PUBLIC HEALTH IN THE 21ST CENTURY SERIES

CROSS INFECTIONS: TYPES, CAUSES AND PREVENTION

AF811424

PUBLIC HEALTH IN THE 21ST CENTURY SERIES

Health-Related Quality of Life
Erik C. Hoffmann (Editor)
2009. ISBN: 978-1-60741-723-1

COPD Is/Is Not a Systemic Disease?
Claudio F. Donner (Editor)
2009. ISBN: 978-1-60876-051-0

Cross Infections: Types, Causes and Prevention
Jin Dong and Xun Liang (Editors)
2009. ISBN: 978-1-60741-467-4

PUBLIC HEALTH IN THE 21ST CENTURY SERIES

CROSS INFECTIONS: TYPES, CAUSES AND PREVENTION

JIN DONG
AND
XUN LIANG
EDITORS

Nova Biomedical Books
New York

Copyright © 2009 by Nova Science Publishers, Inc.

All rights reserved. No part of this book may be reproduced, stored in a retrieval system or transmitted in any form or by any means: electronic, electrostatic, magnetic, tape, mechanical photocopying, recording or otherwise without the written permission of the Publisher.

For permission to use material from this book please contact us:
Telephone 631-231-7269; Fax 631-231-8175
Web Site: http://www.novapublishers.com

NOTICE TO THE READER

The Publisher has taken reasonable care in the preparation of this book, but makes no expressed or implied warranty of any kind and assumes no responsibility for any errors or omissions. No liability is assumed for incidental or consequential damages in connection with or arising out of information contained in this book. The Publisher shall not be liable for any special, consequential, or exemplary damages resulting, in whole or in part, from the readers' use of, or reliance upon, this material. Any parts of this book based on government reports are so indicated and copyright is claimed for those parts to the extent applicable to compilations of such works.

Independent verification should be sought for any data, advice or recommendations contained in this book. In addition, no responsibility is assumed by the publisher for any injury and/or damage to persons or property arising from any methods, products, instructions, ideas or otherwise contained in this publication.

This publication is designed to provide accurate and authoritative information with regard to the subject matter covered herein. It is sold with the clear understanding that the Publisher is not engaged in rendering legal or any other professional services. If legal or any other expert assistance is required, the services of a competent person should be sought. FROM A DECLARATION OF PARTICIPANTS JOINTLY ADOPTED BY A COMMITTEE OF THE AMERICAN BAR ASSOCIATION AND A COMMITTEE OF PUBLISHERS.

Library of Congress Cataloging-in-Publication Data

Cross infections : types, causes and prevention / [edited by] Jin Dong, Xun Liang.
p. ; cm.
Includes bibliographical references and index.
ISBN 978-1-60741-467-4 (hardcover : alk. paper)
1. Nosocomial infections. I. Dong, Jin. II. Liang, Xun.
[DNLM: 1. Cross Infection--prevention & control. 2. Infection Control. WX 167 C951 2009]
RA969.C762 2009
614.4'4--dc22

2009027753

Published by Nova Science Publishers, Inc. ✦ New York

Contents

Preface

Cross infection is the transmission of an infectious agent from one person to another because of a poor barrier protection as in patients and immunocompromised hosts. The most common are nosocomial cross infections, which are acquired at a hospital or other healthcare facilities such as outpatient clinics. This book analyzes infection control for healthcare workers, epidemiologists, administrations and those responsible for infection control programmes at healthcare facilities. Most carriers of infections are unaware of their condition and therefore it is important that prevention of cross-infection routine is adopted for all patients. The prevention of cross transmission of respiratory viral pathogens in pediatric cancer patients with conventional chemotherapy is also explored. Pediatric cancer patients face an increased risk of potentially life-threatening infectious complications due to their underlying malignancy and to the adverse effects of intensive anticancer treatment. This book further delves into the various aspects of catheter-related infections (CRI) such as diagnosis, incidence, etiology, pathogenesis and recommended preventive measures. Other chapters in this book focus on the newly emerging CA-MRSA strains which have caused serious community-acquired infections in otherwise healthy children, an examination of the pathogenesis and microbial properties that contribute to the persistence of S. aureus in dairy cattle herds, a review of the multi-drug resistant pathogens that are common in patients with severe acute exacerbations of chronic obstructive pulmonary disease and a discussion of the microbes which cause cross infections and are resistant to antimicrobial agents, and thus present a challenge in treatment and prevention.

Chapter 1 - This chapter is aimed at infection control for healthcare workers, epidemiologists, administrators, and those responsible for infection control programmes at healthcare facilities. Healthcare delivery from primarily an acute care hospital setting to other healthcare facilities require strategies that can be applied in settings using principles of infection control practice. Standard Precautions has led to a reaffirmation of this approach as the basis for prevention of transmission of infectious agents in these settings. Standard Precautions is a philosophy that considers all patients to be infected with pathogenic organisms hence certain basic infection control procedures must be used during the care of all patients. Body fluids, secretions, excretions and tissues may be contaminated with a variety of different pathogens. Most carriers of infection are unaware of their condition and therefore it is important that prevention of cross-infection routine is adopted for all patients. Routine cross-infection control procedures not only safeguard patients but also protect the healthcare worker. Every member of the medical workforce has a duty to ensure that all necessary precautions are taken to prevent cross-infection to both patients and themselves. The only safe approach is to assume that every patient is a carrier. There is overwhelming evidence that environmental control measures decrease the risk of cross infections in patients, in addition to influences on healthcare personnel infection control practices, and are important factors in preventing transmission of infectious agents. The incidence of hospital acquired infections in all healthcare settings, and the body of knowledge concerning prevention of transmission of these infections has created a need for specific recommendations for the control of these pathogens that would be practical and effective across the continuum of care.

Chapter II - Newly-emerging community-associated methicillin resistant *Staphylococcus aureus* (CA-MRSA) strains have caused serious community-acquired infections in otherwise healthy children, athletes, and young adults lacking typical risk factors for nosocomial MRSA acquisition. The most commonly encountered clinical manifestations include severe skin and soft tissue infections and necrotizing pneumonia. These strains often carry the Panton-Valentine leukocidin (PVL) genes. PVL is a bi-component, pore-forming leukotoxin, recently classified as a member of the family of synergohymenotropic toxins, which causes leukocyte destruction and tissue necrosis but also possesses chemotactic and proinflammatory properties. However, the specific role of PVL as a major virulence factor in CA-MRSA infections has been controversial. Recent studies of PVL knockout strains of CA-MRSA USA300 and USA400 in murine sepsis and abscess models have shown that PVL(-) strains were as lethal and virulent as wild-type strains and caused comparable skin diseases, and that lysis of human neutrophils and pathogen survival after phagocytosis were similar between wild-type and mutant strains. However, a study using a laboratory stain overexpressing plasmid-encoded PVL gene in a mouse acute pneumonia model indicated that PVL alone is sufficient to cause necrotizing pneumonia. But another study using a different murine model of staphylococcal pneumonia that mimics clinicopathologic features of human disease did not support PVL having any impact in this model, and anti-PVL serum failed to protect mice from staphylococcal pneumonia. In addition, recent studies of human CA-MRSA infections in community and hospital patients in the authors' health care region over a six-year period identified the co-existence of two USA400 (a major clonal group of CA-MRSA) sibling strains with and without PVL genes. These strains shared identical genotypic, phenotypic and clinical characteristics. PCR and sequence analysis indicated that the PVL carrying prophage ϕSa2mw was present in PVL(+) but absent in PVL(-) USA400 isolates. These findings provided the first direct human evidence that PVL genes are not necessarily the key determinants associated with the increased dissemination of CA-MRSA strains. The authorsconducted further experimental studies using various in vitro cell culture and animal models of these sibling strains and found that PVL(+) and PVL(-) USA400 strains exhibited identical virulence characteristics in these models. Combined with data from murine models, the weight of the evidence currently suggests that the genomic milieu rather than the PVL gene plays the most significant role in the virulence and widespread dissemination of CA-MRSA.

Chapter III - The advent of intensive care units (ICUs) has led to advances in the treatment of critical-care patients, increasing the survival even of high risk populations such as septic, immunodepressed and oncologic patients and very-low-weight preterm newborns. However, the evolution of the therapeutic arsenal using increasingly more invasive techniques has resulted in the breakdown of barriers and the exposure of previously intact tissues that thus become susceptible to infection. Catheter-related infections (CRI) are one example of this reality and occur when a microorganism invades the bloodstream through a vascular catheter. Infections associated with the use of intravascular devices account for 10 to 20% of all nosocomial infections and are one of the most frequent causes of morbidity and mortality, representing a source of bacteremia and sepsis in hospitalized patients and increasing the length of hospital stay, hospitalization costs and mortality. Approximately 65% of these infections result from the migration of microorganisms of the skin microbiota from the insertion site of the catheter. Intraluminal contamination is observed in 30% of cases and 5% occur through other routes such as infusion of contaminated fluids and distant infectious foci. All of these contamination sources are important, but the most prevalent is contamination with microorganisms of the patient himself in areas close to the insertion site of the catheter. This explains why coagulase-negative staphylococci (CNS) are the microorganisms most frequently associated with this type of infection since they are also the most common in skin. CRI are diagnosed when identical microorganisms are isolated from catheter cultures and from blood cultures in the absence of any apparent source of infection, except for the catheter. The reliability of catheter cultures for the diagnosis of CRI depends on the culture technique used. The objective of this chapter was to review various aspects of CRI such as diagnosis, incidence, etiology, pathogenesis, main recommended preventive measures, use of catheters impregnated with antiseptic, antimicrobial and anticoagulant agents, and new prevention strategies based on the knowledge of the mechanisms of bacterial adhesion and biofilm formation. Biofilm formation is regulated by the exchange of chemical signals between cells during a process called "quorum-sensing". A new approach to prevent the colonization of catheters and to reduce infections related to these devices is to interfere with this cell-cell communication which permits these microorganisms to organize themselves into complex biofilms, protecting them from the host immune system and conferring greater resistance to antimicrobials.

Chapter IV - Today, HAIs are considered to be important adverse outcomes in terms of increased morbidity and mortality, postponed chemotherapy treatment cycles, as well as prolonged duration of hospital stay and additional costs from the perspective of the caregiver. All efforts to prevent HAI and to contain the nosocomial spread of pathogens are critical aspects of patient's safety in the hospital environment. Thus, the prospective surveillance of HAI should be recognized as a fundamental component of quality assurance and control in the treatment of immunocompromised pediatric cancer patients. Pediatric oncologists, pediatric infectious disease specialists, and infection control personnel should combine their efforts and work together improving the quality of supportive care and eliminating the preventable proportion of HAIs in pediatric oncology departments.

Chapter V - In pediatric patients with cancer and intensive chemotherapy viral infections of the respiratory tract (VRTI) may result in life-threatening complications, including infection of the lower respiratory tract (bronchiolitis, pneumonia, acute respiratory failure). Respiratory tract infection of the upper airways may severely compromise breathing (acute airway obstruction) and cause recurrent aspiration in children with brain tumors, with impaired ability to swallow or with a tracheostoma in place.

As a consequence of the chemotherapy-induced suppression of the cellular and the humoral immune response or of the serious immunodeficiency related to the underlying disease (e.g. leukemia, Hodgkin disease) pediatric cancer patients face an increased risk of hematogenous spread of certain viral pathogens from the respiratory tract to other organs as the liver, the bone-marrow and the central nervous system. In addition, atypical manifestations of viral infections in patients, who are not able to mount a sufficient immune response, may prevent an early recognition of the viral etiology of clinical symptoms and in inadequate treatment due to delayed diagnosis.

In a recent study performed in 4 Finnish University Hospitals, Koskenvuo et al. investigated the concomitant presence of 16 viral pathogens in pediatric leukemia patients with blood stream infection (BSI). The prospective evaluation of 156 febrile episodes in 51 children yielded 19 BSI (11%). In 11 of these events (58%) evidence was found for probable concomitant viral infection (5 rhinovirus, 4 respiratory syncytial virus, 2 calicivirus, one enterovirus and one HHV-6 infection). In a previous study from Turku, Finland, microbiologically confirmed respiratory virus infections were found in 28 of 75 (37%) consecutive febrile episodes in 32 children during anticancer treatment. In this clinical setting, viral infection may per se cause severe clinical symptoms or may pave the way for bacterial infections like pneumonia or BSI.

From these studies it can be concluded that there is a diagnostic gap considering viral etiologies in pediatric cancer patients with 'fever of unknown origin' due to insufficient efforts to diagnose these events in clinical practice.

The epidemiology and treatment of viral respiratory tract infections in patients, who have received a stem cell transplant, has recently been extensively reviewed in excellent articles. This chapter focuses on the prevention of cross transmission of respiratory viral pathogens in pediatric cancer patients with conventional chemotherapy.

Chapter VI - Mastitis is an infectious disease that is highly prevalent in dairy herds and responsible for financial losses worldwide. Most losses are attributed to subclinical mastitis, which is only detectable with indirect diagnostic tests using milk samples. *Staphylococcus aureus* is the main causative agent of mastitis in dairy herds. The udder of infected cows is the main reservoir of *S. aureus*, which can be transmitted to other cows in the herd. There are numerous sources of *S. aureus*, including stables and feeds, equipment and animal skin of cattle and other species, as well as humans themselves. Teat skin has been implicated as an important reservoir for intramammary infection; however, transmission from man has been proposed. Various virulence factors are responsible for the symptoms and severity of infections caused by *S. aureus*. These factors include hemolysins, leukocidins and a group of toxic pyrogenic superantigens consisting of the toxic shock syndrome toxin 1 (TSST-1) and staphylococcal enterotoxins, which cause staphylococcal food intoxication. *S. aureus* enterotoxins are the most frequent cause of food intoxication, with reports of cases due to food manipulation after heat treatment. Heat destroys the vegetative bacterial microbiota in food, and non-competitive staphylococci, introduced by inadequate manipulation, may grow. Food intoxication is the result of the ingestion of foods contaminated with enterotoxigenic *S. aureus* during or after processing, inappropriate management or even inadequate refrigeration, enabling the growth of microorganisms and the production and release of toxins into the food which, when ingested, will produce all characteristic signs and symptoms. Staphylococcal enterotoxins are primarily found in foods that contain proteins and carbohydrates, such as dairy products, pastries, processed meat, mayonnaise, and salads. Inadequate manipulation of the product may increase the population of staphylococci until the time of pasteurization, implying the possibility of production of enterotoxins that are stable at high temperatures. Thus, pasteurized milk would be free of microorganisms, but not of enterotoxins. This milk may subsequently be offered to children who depend on it for their growth, a fact representing a serious public health problem. The objective of this chapter is to provide data for a better understanding of the pathogenesis and microbial properties that contribute to the persistence of *S. aureus* in dairy cattle herds.

Chapter VII - Severe acute exacerbations of chronic obstructive pulmonary disease requiring mechanical ventilation are frequently attributed to bacteria. Multi-drug resistant pathogens are common in patients with severe acute exacerbations of chronic obstructive pulmonary disease, especially when they were previously intubated or had used antibiotics. These pathogens are also associated with increased rate of initially inappropriate antibiotic therapy. Although multi-drug resistant bacteria are not independently associated with increased intensive care unit mortality, an initially inappropriate antibiotic treatment is an independent factor for intensive care unit mortality in patients with severe acute exacerbations of chronic obstructive epulmonary disease. This may be explained by the higher ventilator-associated pneumonia rates observed in these patients Ventilator-associated pneumonia is independently associated with increased intensive care unit mortality in patients with severe acute exacerbations of chronic obstructive pulmonary disease. Therefore, for mechanically ventilated patients with severe acute exacerbations of chronic obstructive pulmonary disease an initially appropriate antibiotic regimen might have beneficial impact on clinical outcomes. Given the growing antimicrobial resistance for *Streptococcus pneumoniae* and the high incidence of β-lactamase producing strains, penicillin's and macrolides may not be appropriate, whereas *Pseudomonas aeruginosa* and *Stenotrophomonas* species and therefor broad spectrum antibiotics should probably be considered. However, although an initially broad spectrum antibiotic regimen might be reasonable, there is limited evidence to support that it would improve outcomes. Therefore, the data available advise that an initially appropriate empiric antimicrobial regimen should largely rely on local microbiology and routine microbial investigations, to control for unexpected or resistant pathogens. This approach may increase the rates of an initially appropriate antimicrobial regimen, until solid evidence become available regarding the potential role of broad spectrum empiric antibiotics in severe acute exacerbations of chronic obstructive pulmonary disease requiring mechanical ventilation

Chapter VIII - Epidemiological surveillance is an essential element of any infection control programme, especially in intensive care units (ICUs), to increase awareness and to identify areas for improvement. The majority of healthcare-associated infections (HAI) is of endogenous origin and therefore difficult to prevent. In contrast, exogenous infections are more likely to be preventable by standard or specific precautions devised to reduce the overall rates of nosocomial transmission. To demonstrate the exogenous route of infection, the use of highly discriminatory typing techniques is necessary: undistinguishable strains isolated from different patients may indicate that cross-transmission from one patient to another has occurred. Different methodological approaches can be used to estimate the preventable proportion of HAI. Most of the studies are laboratory driven and did not include a daily follow-up of patient status. Ideally, integrating laboratory data with active surveillance, would provide systematic observations and measurement of infection events, as well as clonality data [Scheckler et al., 1998; Agodi and Pasquarella, 2000; Agodi A, 2000]. One such approach consists in the assessment of the preventable proportion of infections integrating clonality assessment with a unit-based surveillance protocol intended for continuous surveillance, in which denominator data (patient-days) are collected for the entire unit. Although indicators generated by such a 'first-level' surveillance are not suitable for ICU benchmarking of quality of care in terms of infection control, they are appropriate for the follow-up of infections within the same unit and for regional, national and international investigation of trends for pathogen-specific infection rates. This approach has been used in a study conducted with the main aim to investigate the epidemiological impact of *Acinetobacter baumannii* HAI in a Sicilian ICU and to estimate the preventable proportion of *Acinetobacter* infections, i.e., those resulting from cross-transmission [Agodi et al., 2006].

An alternative comprehensive approach integrating the patient-based surveillance data, intended for advanced risk-adjusted comparison of infection rates between ICUs, with molecular typing data has been adopted in a recent study in order to investigate the clonality patterns sustaining the endemic *versus* the epidemic mode of transmission for acquisition of the three emerging multiresistant pathogens, *Pseudomonas aeruginosa*, *A. baumannii* and *Stenotrophomonas maltophilia*.

The present survey provides a framework for further investigation of the role of alert pathogens and/or high-risk clones together with patients' risk factor profiles for appropriate design of effective control strategies especially addressed to ICU patients.

Chapter IX - Still in the era of potent, combined antiretroviral therapy, late recognition of HIV disease or lack of sufficient immune recovery pose HIV-infected patients at risk to develop opportunistic infections by atypical mycobacteria, which are environmental organisms commonly retrieved in soil and superficial waters. Among these microorganisms, the most frequent is represented by Mycobacterium avium-intracellulare (Mycobacterium avium-intracellulare complex, or MAC). Health care professionals who face HIV-infected patients should suspect disseminated mycobacterial disease when a deep immunodeficiency is present, as represented by a CD4+ lymphocyte count below 50-100 cells/μL, and often systemic, non-specific signs and symptoms, and associated non-specific laboratory abnormalities. Mycobacterial culture of peripheral blood is a reliable technique for diagnosing disseminated disease. A set of two cultures may identify over 95% of cases of Mycobacterium avium-intracellulare bacteremia. Microscopical examination (Ziehl-Nielsen stain and comparable techniques), and culture biopsies from other normally sterile body sites (i.e. bone marrow, lymph nodes, or liver), also may be useful to pose a diagnosis of AIDS-related mycobacterial disease. Among drugs active against atypical mycobacteria, besides some anti-tubercular compound, the rifampicin derivative rifabutin, and the novel fluoroquinolones, the availability of macrolides greatly contributed to improve both prophylaxis and treatment outcome of disseminated mycobacteriosis complicating the course of AIDS. Although multiple questions remain about which regimens are optimal, general recommendations can be expressed on the ground of existing evidences. Treatment should begin with associated clarithromycin (or azithromycin), plus ethambutol and rifabutin (with the rifabutin dosing depending on other concomitant medications that might result in drug-drug interactions). A combined three-drug regimen is preferred for patients who cannot be prescribed an effective antiretroviral regimen immediately. Patients with a CD4+ lymphocyte count below 50 cells/μL who do not have clinical evidence of active mycobacterial disease, should receive a primary prophylaxis with either clarithromycin or azithromycin; the latter could be coadministered rifabutin. Anti-mycobacterial prophylaxis may be discontinued in patients without a history of recognized mycobacterial disease, whose CD4+ lymphocyte count remains above 100 cells/μL, for at least three months while on combined antiretroviral therapy. With regard to subjects on secondary antimycobacterial prophylaxis, in appears safe to discontinue it when a sustained CD4+ lymphocyte count exceeds at least 100 cells/μL for at least 3-6 consecutive months, during a concurrent, effective antiretroviral regimen.

Commentary - Cross Infection Control (CIC) is a term that encompasses all the measures taken to prevent the transfer of pathogenic microorganisms, which can potentially result in infection. Control of cross infections in a hospital, outpatient clinic, or a community setting is crucial, especially for immunocompromised patients, such as cancer patients and drug addicts. Unfortunately, the chain of cross infection control is easily broken when simple procedures are not observed.

In: Cross Infections: Types, Causes and Prevention
Editors: Jin Dong and Xun Liang
ISBN: 978-1-60741-467-4
© 2009 Nova Science Publishers, Inc.

Chapter I

Cross Infections

Dushyant Maharaj*
Department of Obstetrics and Gynecology, University of Otago,
Wellington, New Zealand
Consultant, Wellington Women's Hospital, Wellington, New Zealand

Abstract

This chapter is aimed at infection control for healthcare workers, epidemiologists, administrators, and those responsible for infection control programmes at healthcare facilities. Healthcare delivery from primarily an acute care hospital setting to other healthcare facilities require strategies that can be applied in settings using principles of infection control practice. Standard Precautions has led to a reaffirmation of this approach as the basis for prevention of transmission of infectious agents in these settings. Standard Precautions is a philosophy that considers all patients to be infected with pathogenic organisms hence certain basic infection control procedures must be used during the care of all patients. Body fluids, secretions, excretions and tissues may be contaminated with a variety of different pathogens. Most carriers of infection are unaware of their condition and therefore it is important that prevention of cross-infection routine is adopted for all patients. Routine cross-infection control procedures not only safeguard patients but also protect the healthcare worker. Every member of the medical workforce has a duty to ensure that all necessary precautions are taken to prevent cross-infection to both patients and themselves. The only safe approach is to assume that every patient is a carrier. There is overwhelming evidence that environmental control measures decrease the risk of cross infections in patients, in addition to influences on healthcare personnel infection control practices, and are important factors in preventing transmission of infectious agents. The incidence of hospital acquired infections in all healthcare settings, and the body of knowledge concerning prevention of transmission of these infections has created a need for specific recommendations for the control of these pathogens that would be practical and effective across the continuum of care.

* Corresponding Author: PO Box 7343 Wellington South 6242 Wellington New Zealand Telephone: +64 4 385 5999 Fax: +64 4 389 5943 e-mail: dean.maharaj@otago.ac.nz

Introduction

Cross infection refers to the transmission of a pathogenic organism from one person to another. It is a common and important mode of infection with a variety of organisms which include bacterial, viral and fungal infections, and parasitic infestations. Cross infection can occur in hospitals, kindergartens, day-care centers, schools, prisons, military barracks, places of employment, and other settings where individuals and groups interact with one other. When it happens in a medical setting, such as a hospital or nursing home, it is called nosocomial infection. Nosocomial infections may also be acquired in other ways, such as through hospital staff or inadequately sterilized surgical instruments. Cross infection is a potential problem in all institutional settings, and is an important threat to patient safety [1]. It is important to observe procedures that can minimize this type of infection and limit the effects. These procedures include constant surveillance, maintenance of sanitary conditions, and prompt intervention whenever an infection is detected. The best way to prevent cross infections is by rigorous observance of personal hygiene at all times, and through the use of barrier nursing, sanitary practices, and other pertinent procedures termed "*standard precautions*". Standard Precautions are work practices implemented to achieve a basic standard of infection control in order to minimize cross infection. These precautions can reduce the potential for transmission of infection from person to person, whether patient, nursing, medical or allied health or staff member. Standard precautions combine the major features of universal precautions and body substance isolation. The term "body substance isolation" focuses on protecting patients and health personnel from all moist and potentially infected body substances (secretions and excretions), not just blood. "Transmission based precautions" are recommended when a patient is known to be, or is suspected of being infected or colonized with pathogens which are epidemiologically important, for example, antibiotic resistant organisms or those easily spread – such as by airborne or droplet transmission. These precautions underpin routine safe practice, protecting both staff and clients from infection. By applying standard precautions at all times, and to all patients, best practice becomes second nature and the risks of infection are minimised. Lack of adherence to established standards and guidance can result in adverse patient outcomes in health-care facilities [2]. The principles underlying standard precautions include [3]:

1. achieving optimum hand hygiene
2. using personal protective equipment
3. safe handling and disposal of sharps
4. safe handling and disposal of clinical waste
5. managing blood and bodily fluids
6. decontaminating equipment
7. achieving and maintaining a clean clinical environment
8. appropriate use of indwelling devices
9. managing accidents
10. good communication – with other health care workers, patients and visitors
11. training/education

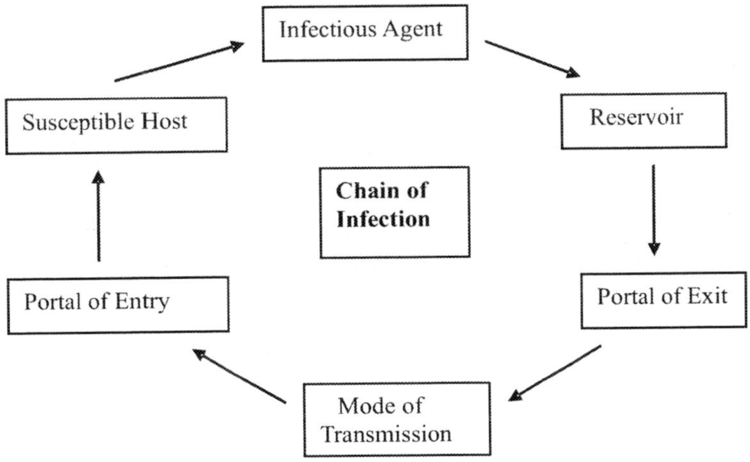

Figure 1. Chain of infection.

Although the environment serves as a reservoir for a variety of microorganisms, it is rarely implicated in disease transmission except in the immunocompromised population. Inadvertent exposures to environmental opportunistic or airborne pathogens may result in infections with significant morbidity and/or mortality. The health-care environment contains a diverse population of microorganisms, but only a few are significant pathogens for susceptible humans. Microorganisms are present in great numbers in moist, organic environments, but some also persist under dry conditions, and assessing their role in causing infection and disease is difficult [4]. Further, the presence of the pathogen does not establish its causal role; its transmission from source to host could be through indirect means, such as hand transferal [4]. The presence of the susceptible host is one of the components of the "*chain of infection*," that underscores the importance of the health-care environment and opportunistic pathogens (Figure 1).

The chain of infection is a circle of links, each representing a component in the cycle. Each link *must* be present and in sequential order for an infection to occur. The links are: infectious agent, reservoir, portal of exit from the reservoir, mode of transmission, and portal of entry into a susceptible host. As a result of advances in medical technology and therapies, more patients are becoming immunocompromised in the course of treatment, and are at increased risk for acquiring health-care-associated opportunistic infections. Trends in health-care delivery, such as early discharge of patients from acute care facilities also are changing the distribution of patient populations and increasing the number of immunocompromised persons in non-acute-care hospitals. Those patients remaining in acute-care facilities are likely to be those requiring extensive medical interventions and are at higher risk for opportunistic infection [2].

In some areas of practice, such as obstetrics, with the advent of antibiotics and a change in the virulence of organisms responsible for lethal infection, namely group A hemolytic streptococcus, the emphasis has shifted away from infections due to microbes. There has been a shift to another generation of pathogenic micro-organisms, mostly viral. Some of these are transmissible in the health-care setting between attendants and patients as well as among patients. Although there are certain features in common, there are notable differences in the biological behavior, infectivity, and methods of transmission between viruses and microbes.

The impact of viral infections, accompanied by greater understanding of their virulence, infectivity, routes of transmission, and natural history has led to significant changes in the measure of care. Examples have been hepatitis B and human immunodeficiency virus (HIV). Transmission of hepatitis B via contaminated serum, and contaminated needles, was well recognized, but it was some time before it was appreciated that this disease was also transmissible via sexual intercourse, and furthermore, it was the explosion of intravenous drug abuse which caused the disorder to attain enhanced social significance [5]. It is now recognized that hepatitis B could be transmitted from surgeon to patient [6]. The transmission rate was approximately 10% after major surgical operations, with infectivity of hepatitis B after accidental inoculation in the order of 20% [5]. It has been proven that hepatitis B virus can be spread in either direction between health-care professionals and patients; because the reverse is also true, this has led to the extension of barrier nursing to cover a number of procedural activities, including surgery and childbirth. HIV infection in obstetrics and gynecology has followed a remarkably similar course. Longitudinal studies have indicated that the vertical transmission rate is of the order of 15%, at least in the asymptomatic phases of the disease [7]. As HIV is known to be spread in much the same manner as hepatitis B virus, it was only a matter of time before evidence was obtained of transmission in the health-care setting [8]. Reported pooled data on percutaneous injuries, revealed a seroconversion rate of approximately 1 in 300 [9]. While there is constant vigilance for HIV-positive patients, infection of patients by HIV seropositive health-care workers has also been documented [10].

Susceptible Hosts

Infection is the result of a complex interrelationship between a host and an infectious agent. Factors that influence infection include the occurrence and severity of disease, characteristics of the host-agent interaction, virulence and antigenicity of the organism, the infectious dose, mechanisms of disease evolution, and route of exposure [11]. Outcomes following exposure to an infectious agent vary amongst individuals. Not all individuals exposed to pathogenic microorganisms develop symptomatic disease, yet others become severely ill, and may even die after a relatively minor exposure. Others may become transiently or permanently colonized but remain asymptomatic, while others progress from colonization to symptomatic disease, either immediately following exposure, or after a period of asymptomatic colonization. Immunity at the time of exposure to an infectious agent, interaction between pathogens, and virulence intrinsic to the agent are important predictors of an individuals' response to infections. Host factors such as extremes of age and underlying disease, HIV/acquired immune deficiency syndrome (AIDS), and malignancy can increase susceptibility to infection. A variety of medications that alter the normal flora (e.g., antimicrobial agents, gastric acid suppressants, corticosteroids, anti-rejection drugs, anti-neoplastic agents, and immunosuppressive drugs can also increase susceptibility to infections [12,13,14,15,16,17]. Surgical procedures and radiation therapy also impair defenses of organ systems. Indwelling devices such as urinary catheters, endotracheal tubes, central venous and arterial lines and synthetic implants facilitate development of infections by allowing potential pathogens to bypass local defenses that would ordinarily impede their invasion, and by providing surfaces for development of biofilms that may facilitate adherence of microorganisms and protect from antimicrobial activity [18,19,20]. Some infections associated with invasive procedures result from transmission within the healthcare facility; while others arise from the patient's endogenous flora [21,22,23,24,25].

Modes of Transmission

Several classes of pathogens can cause infection, including bacteria, viruses, fungi, parasites, and prions. The modes of transmission vary by type of organism; while some infectious agents may be transmitted by more than one route, others are transmitted primarily by direct or indirect contact, (e.g., *Herpes simplex* virus [HSV], respiratory syncytial virus, *Staphylococcus aureus*), others by droplet, (e.g., influenza virus, *B. pertussis*) or airborne routes (e.g., *M. tuberculosis).* Other infectious agents, such as bloodborne viruses (e.g., hepatitis B and C viruses [HBV, HCV] and HIV are transmitted rarely via percutaneous or mucous membrane exposure. Importantly, not all infectious agents are transmitted from person to person.

Contact Transmission

Contact transmission is the most common mode of transmission, and is divided into two subgroups: direct contact and indirect contact. Direct transmission occurs when micro-organisms are transferred from one infected person to another without a contaminated intermediate object or person. Direct contact transmission between patients and healthcare personnel include:

- blood or other body fluids from a patient directly enters a caregiver's body through contact with a mucous membrane or breaks, such as cuts and abrasions in the skin [26,27].
- mites from a scabies-infested patient are transferred to the skin of a caregiver while having direct ungloved contact with the patient's skin [28,29].
- a healthcare provider may develop herpetic lesions on a finger after contact with HSV without using gloves [30,31]

Indirect transmission involves the transfer of an infectious agent through a contaminated intermediate object or fomite, or person. A "fomite"is an inanimate object, which in itself is not harmful, but is able to harbor pathogenic micro-organisms and thus may serve as an agent for transmission of infection. The contaminated hands of healthcare personnel are important contributors to indirect contact transmission [32]. Examples of opportunities for indirect contact transmission include:

- Hands of healthcare personnel, after touching an infected body site of a patient or a fomite [33,34].
- Patient-care devices (e.g.,thermometers) may transmit pathogens if devices are shared between patients without cleaning and disinfecting between patients [35,36].

- Shared toys may become a vehicle for transmitting respiratory viruses among pediatric patients [37, 38].
- Instruments that are inadequately cleaned between patients before disinfection or sterilization [39,40, 41].
- Contaminated clothing, uniforms, laboratory coats, or gowns used as personal protective equipment, have the potential to colonize or infect a patient with an infectious agent [42,43].

Droplet Transmission

Some infectious agents may be transmitted by the droplet route, either directly or indirectly. Droplets traditionally have been defined as being >5 μm in size. Respiratory droplets carrying infectious pathogens transmit infection when they travel directly from the respiratory tract of the infected individual to a susceptible recipient. The droplets are generated when an infected person coughs, sneezes, or talks, or during procedures such as suctioning, endotracheal intubation, cough induction by chest physiotherapy, and during cardiopulmonary resuscitation [44,45,46,47,48,49]. Studies have shown that the nasal mucosa, conjunctivae and less frequently the mouth, are susceptible portals of entry for respiratory viruses [50]. The maximum distance for droplet transmission has historically been the area of defined risk, arbitrarily set at a distance of less than 3 feet around the patient [51,52]. The distance droplets travel depends on the velocity and mechanism by which they are propelled from the source, the density of respiratory secretions, environmental temperature and humidity, and the ability of the pathogen to maintain infectivity over a distance [53]. A distance of less than 3 feet around the patient is arbitrary chosen, and should not be used as the sole criterion for deciding when a mask should be worn to protect oneself from droplet exposure. It may therefore be prudent to don a mask when within 6 to 10 feet of the patient, or upon entry into the patient's room. Droplet nuclei, defined as particles <5 μm in size arising from desiccation of suspended droplets, have also been associated with airborne transmission [53]. A range of droplet sizes, including those with diameters of 30μm or greater, can remain suspended in the air, and are able to remain infective [54]. Examples of infectious agents that are transmitted via the droplet route include *Bordetella pertussis*, influenza virus, adenovirus, rhinovirus, *Mycoplasma pneumoniae*, SARS-associated coronavirus, group A streptococcus, and *Neisseria meningitidis*.

Airborne Transmission

Airborne transmission occurs by dissemination of either airborne droplet nuclei or small particles containing infectious agents that remain infective over time and distance (e.g., *Mycobacterium tuberculosis*). Microorganisms carried in this manner may be dispersed over long distances by air currents and may be inhaled by susceptible individuals who have not had direct contact with the infectious individual [55,56,57]. For certain other respiratory infectious agents, such as influenza and rhinovirus, and even some gastrointestinal viruses, there is evidence that the pathogen may be transmitted via small-particle aerosols [58,59,60,61].

Transmission from Patients

Airborne transmission over a limited distance (e.g. within a room), has been suggested as the route for transmission of infectious agents such as influenza virus and noroviruses [58,62,63]. Although the most frequent routes of transmission of noroviruses are contact and food and waterborne routes, reports suggest that noroviruses may be transmitted through aerosolization of infectious particles from vomitus or fecal material which are inhaled and subsequently swallowed [62,63].

Transmission from the Environment

Some airborne infectious agents are derived from the environment and do not usually involve person-to-person transmission. For example, anthrax spores can be aerosolized from contaminated environmental surfaces and inhaled into the respiratory tract [64,65]. Spores of environmental fungi, such as *Aspergillus* are widespread in the environment and may cause infections in immunocompromised patients who inhale these spores [66,67].

Other Sources of Infection

Transmission of infection from sources other than infectious individuals, include common environmental sources or vehicles, such as contaminated food, water, or medications (e.g. intravenous fluids). *Vectorborne transmission* of infectious agents from mosquitoes, flies, rats, and other vermin also can occur in healthcare settings [68].

Transmission Risks in Healthcare Settings

Factors that influence differences in transmission risks among the various healthcare settings include the population characteristics, such as age and increased susceptibility to infections, intensity of care, exposure to environmental sources, length of stay in a facility, and frequency of interaction between patients/residents with each other and with healthcare workers. In addition, organizational priorities, goals, and resources influence how different healthcare settings meet their specific needs [69,70]. Infection control management decisions are informed by data regarding institutional experience and epidemiology, trends, and emerging infectious disease threats [68]. If transmission in outpatient settings is to be prevented, screening for potentially infectious individuals, especially those who may be at risk for transmitting airborne infectious agents, is necessary at the initial patient encounter. Once a potentially infectious patient has been identified, implementation of prevention measures, such as prompt separation of the patient and implementation of appropriate control measures can decrease transmission risks [71,72].

Hospitals

Cross infections risks are present in all hospital settings. Certain settings and patient populations have unique conditions that predispose patients to infection. These are often sentinel sites for the emergence of new transmission risks that may be unique to that setting, or present opportunities for transmission to other settings in the hospital.

Intensive Care Units

Intensive care units (ICUs) serve patients who are in a moribund state, such as those with major trauma, respiratory failure and other life-threatening conditions. Although ICUs account for a relatively small proportion of hospitalized patients, infections acquired in these units accounted for >20% of all hospital acquired infections [73]. This patient population has increased susceptibility to colonization and infection because of underlying morbidity, invasive medical devices and technology used in their care, the high frequency of contact with healthcare personnel, prolonged stay, and prolonged exposure to antimicrobial agents [74,75,76]. Outbreaks associated with a variety of bacterial, fungal and viral pathogens due to common source and person-to-person transmissions are frequent in the ICU setting [77,78,79].

Burn Units

Wounds following burns can provide fertile conditions for colonization, infection, and transmission of pathogens. In patients with a burn injury involving >30% of the total body surface area, the risk of infection is particularly high [80,81]. Staphylococcus aureus, enterococci, gram-negative bacteria, and candida are prevalent pathogens in burn infections [82,83,84,85,86,87]. Advances in burn care, namely, early excision and grafting of the burn wound, use of topical antimicrobials, early enteral feeding, prophylactic antimicrobial usage, selective digestive decontamination, and use of antimicrobial-coated catheters have led to decreased infectious complications. Despite these advances, there is no consensus on the most effective infection control practices to prevent transmission of infections in patients with serious burns. There also is controversy regarding the need for and type of barrier precautions for routine care of burn patients [68,88].

Pediatrics

The most outstanding advances in provision of neonatal care have arisen from the capacity of neonatologists to provide the potential for survival of infants of ever-decreasing size and gestational age. The median neonatal survival is now to be found at around 25-26 weeks of gestational age, a concept which was unthinkable two decades ago [89]. These successes have wrought other problems for very small neonates, often of an infective nature. Organisms that are ordinarily commensals assume a pathogenic status with sometimes lethal outcomes. The most obvious of these is group B haemolytic streptococcus, but there are other organisms which can have a similar devastating effect in a neonatal nursery. A swing of the pendulum back towards tighter infection control procedures in the perinatal period has been instituted as a result of the influence of neonatal paediatricians [5]. The epidemiology of hospital acquired infections in children identified unique issues peculiar to this group of hospitalized patients [90,91,92]. Neonatal intensive care unit (NICU) patients and the low birthweight babies had high rates of central venous catheter-associated bloodstream infections [93, 94].

Besides neonates acquiring infections, staff in attendance at deliveries, and those involved in neonatal resuscitation and care must protect themselves against potential infections a neonate may have acquired from the mother. The newly delivered infant must be regarded as contaminated until cleaned of blood and amniotic fluid. The important principle is that until the infant is cleaned, it must be handled as if contaminated. Utmost vigilance should be exercised during cord blood sampling and handling of the secundines for examination and disposal. The insertion of a needle into umbilical cord held between two fingers is fraught with danger and should be forbidden. The cord can be steadied between sponge holders and samples can be withdrawn from vessels on the fetal surface of the placenta. Further procedural difficulties arise from the fact that the collector of the blood is almost always wearing contaminated gloves at the time when this procedure is carried out. Unless there is another individual immediately at hand with appropriate equipment, the outside of the receptacle for the blood will almost always be contaminated and this presents a theoretical hazard to the laboratory staff. Desirable practice would be the prior arrangement of the appropriate receptacles, with removal of their caps and placement in an appropriate rack to prevent tipping over [5].

In the older pediatric age there is a high prevalence of community-acquired infections among hospitalized children who have not yet become immune either by vaccination or by naturally acquired infection. The result is that more patients with transmissible infections present in pediatric healthcare settings, especially during seasonal epidemics of respiratory infections, measles, chickenpox, and rotavirus [68].Close physical contact between healthcare workers and children provide opportunities for transmission of infections. The congregation of children in playareas, where toys and bodily secretions are easily shared, and family members rooming-in with pediatric patients can further increase the risk of transmission [95]. In addition, several other factors may increase the likelihood of acquiring infection in healthcare settings; immaturity of the neonatal immune system, lack of natural infection and immunity, prevalence of patients with immune deficiencies, congenital anatomic anomalies, and use of invasive devices [96].

Non-Acute Healthcare Settings

In recent times, healthcare is also provided in settings outside of hospitals including, nursing homes, homes for the disabled, behavioral facilities, rehabilitation centers and hospices [97]. In addition, healthcare may be provided in settings such as occupational health clinics in workplaces, adult day care centers, homeless shelters, prisons, school clinics and infirmaries. Each of these settings has risks to consider when designing and implementing an infection control program. Facilities other than primary healthcare settings in which healthcare may be delivered include correctional facilities and shelters for the homeless. Both settings can have crowded conditions and poor ventilation. Indigent individuals who may have chronic illnesses, alcoholism, drug use, poor nutrition, or the homeless, often receive their primary healthcare at sites such as these [98]. Infectious diseases under these circumstances include tuberculosis, scabies, respiratory infections, sexually transmitted and bloodborne diseases, hepatitis A virus, and diarrheal pathogens [99,100,101]. Patient encounters in sites such as correctional facilities and shelters for the homeless provide an opportunity to deliver immunizations and screening for *M. tuberculosis* infection in addition to diagnosing and treating acute illnesses [102]. Recommended infection control measures in these non-traditional areas designated for healthcare delivery are the same as for other ambulatory care settings. Continued compliance with infection control measures will decrease the risk of health-care–associated infections among patients, especially the immunocompromised, and health-care workers.

Estimates of acquired infection rates of 1.8 to 13.5 per 1000 resident-care days have been reported in some of these facilities [103,104]. Since residents interact freely with each other, controlling transmission of infection in nursing home settings can be a challenge [105]. Those who are colonized or infected with certain microorganisms are, in some cases, restricted to their room, however, because of the psychosocial risks associated with such restriction it is recommended that their psychosocial needs be balanced with infection control needs [106]. Risk factors for infection among nursing home residents include an age-related decline in immunity, increased susceptibility to infections, immobility, incontinence, underlying chronic diseases, poor functional status, and malnutrition [107,108,109]. Certain medications that affect an individual's level of consciousness, immune function, gastric acid secretions, normal flora, as well as the use of invasive devices, increase susceptibility to infection and colonization in nursing home residents [110,111]. Outbreaks of infections in these facilities can lead to substantial morbidity and mortality, and increased medical costs. Finally, limited functional status and total dependence on healthcare personnel for day-to-day activities have been identified as independent risk factors for infection and colonization with certain pathogens [112,113]. Because residents of nursing homes and pediatric rehabilitation units are hospitalized frequently, they can transfer pathogens between their residence and hospitals [114,115,116,117].

Ambulatory Care

In the recent past, healthcare delivery in many countries has shifted from the hospital inpatient to ambulatory and community-based settings, including home-care. Ambulatory care is provided in clinics, physician offices, dialysis centers, surgical centers, and many others. This form of care now accounts for most patient encounters with the health care system [118]. In these settings, adapting transmission prevention guidelines is challenging because patients remain in common rooms for prolonged periods waiting to be seen, or awaiting admission to the hospital, examination rooms are turned around quickly with limited cleaning, and infectious patients may not be identified [68].

Transmission of bloodborne pathogens may occur in healthcare settings usually from contaminated medical devices, multi-dose vials, or intravenous solutions [119,120]. These cases have invariably been attributed to failure to adhere to basic infection control principles, such as safe injection practices and aseptic technique [121]. Transmission of various pathogens via incompletely disinfected equipment, healthcare workers to patients, and patient-to-patient in ambulatory settings has been reported [122,123,124,125].

Prevention of Transmission of Infectious Agents in Healthcare Settings

Administrative Measures

Healthcare organizations should commit to preventing transmission of infectious agents by incorporating infection control into the objectives of the organization's patient and occupational safety programs [126,127,128]. An institutional system to guide, support, and monitor adherence to infection control precautions and measures will facilitate the organization's mission, commitment, and achievement in decreasing hospital acquired infections [129,130]. Policies and procedures should be in place, and regularly updated to ensure the success of these measures. A key administrative measure is provision of financial and human resources for maintaining infection control, and occupational health programs that are responsive to emerging needs. Specific components include staffing levels, construction and design decisions, microbiology laboratory support, adequate supplies and equipment, including facility ventilation systems, adherence to monitoring, assessment and correction of system failures that contribute to transmission, and provision of feedback to healthcare personnel and senior administrators [68]. Other administrative factors that affect the transmission of infectious agents in healthcare settings include institutional culture, worker behavior, and the work environment. Each of these areas is suitable for performance improvement monitoring and incorporation into the organization's patient safety goals [128,131].

Studies showed that the most effective infection control programs were those that involved a trained infection control physician or microbiologist, and at least one infection control nurse per 250 beds [132].However, in more recent times, there is agreement that infection control staffing can no longer be based on staff-patient ratios alone, but should be determined by the scope of the program, characteristics of the patient population, complexity of the healthcare system, tools available to assist personnel to perform essential tasks, and the needs of the institution and community [133,134,135].

Bedside Nursing Staff

There is evidence that the level of bedside nurse-staffing influences the quality of patient care [136]. If there is adequate nursing staff, it is more likely that infection control practices will be adhered to, and infection rates will decline [137,138,139]. Designating a nurse on a patient care unit as an infection control link nurse is an effective adjunct to enhance infection control at the unit level [140,141]. These individuals should receive training in basic infection control and liase with infection control personnel, but maintain their primary role as bedside nurses. They increase the awareness of infection control protocols and interventions at the unit level.

Laboratory Support Staff

The critical role of the clinical microbiology laboratory in infection control and healthcare epidemiology contributes to preventing transmission of infectious diseases in healthcare settings by detecting and reporting epidemiologically important organisms, identifying emerging patterns of antimicrobial resistance, and assisting in assessment of the effectiveness of protocols to limit transmission during outbreaks [142,143].

Healthcare facilities need to ensure the availability of quality laboratory services, appropriately trained laboratory staff, and systems to promptly communicate epidemiologically important results to those involved in healthcare [144].

Adherence to Guidelines

Studies have shown that adherence to recommended infection control practices decreases transmission of infectious agents in healthcare settings [145,146]. While this is commendable in reducing cross infections, several observational studies have shown limited compliance to recommended practices by healthcare personnel, ranging from 43% to 89% [146,147,148,149, 150,151]. Education to improve compliance with recommended practices is paramount to staff's changes in knowledge and attitude [146,152,153].

Education

Education and training of healthcare personnel are important for ensuring that policies, protocol and procedures are understood and put into practice. Education about the important role of vaccines in protecting healthcare staff, patients, and family members can help improve vaccination rates [154,155]. Education on the principles and practices for preventing transmission of infectious agents should begin in the training years of health professions. In healthcare facilities, education and training should be provided at the time of orientation and be repeated as necessary to maintain competency. Further education and training are necessary when policies and procedures are revised or when there are special circumstances, such as an outbreak of infection. Information about hand hygiene, respiratory hygiene/cough etiquette, vaccination and other standard infection prevention strategies may be incorporated into patient information materials provided upon admission to the healthcare facility. Such information may be helpful in the home environment where household members often have responsibility for adherence to recommended infection control practices [68].

Hand Hygiene

Hand hygiene has been cited frequently as the single most important practice to reduce the transmission of infectious agents in healthcare settings and is an essential element of Standard Precautions [156,157]. The concept of cleansing hands with an antiseptic agent emerged in the early 19th century. In 1822, a French pharmacist demonstrated that solutions containing chlorides of lime or soda could eradicate the foul odors associated with human corpses, and that such solutions could be used as disinfectants and antiseptics [158]. For centuries puerperal infection has been one of the chief causes of morbidity and mortality in the parturient woman. History tells us that Ignaz Semmelweis was the first to recognize the importance of hand washing to prevent cross-contamination of patients, and that it was he who discovered the cause of puerperal or childbed fever [159]. As a 28-year-old assistant physician in the maternity unit of the Vienna General Hospital in the 1840s, Semmelweiss was given the responsibility of examining obstetric patients, supervising difficult deliveries, and organizing teaching rounds both in the morgue and in the first section of the clinical ward, the section in which most deliveries were done by medical students. Semmelweiss realized that the rate of puerperal fever was much higher in the first section than in the second section of the maternity ward, where most of the deliveries were done by nurse-midwives. He also observed that the clinical symptoms of puerperal fever were identical to those of a hospital pathologist, Jakob Kolletschka, who died after pricking his finger with a dirty autopsy instrument. Semmelweiss concluded that the disease was caused by "cadaverous particles" and other decaying organic matter transmitted to the patients in the first section by medical students who arrived on the maternity wards fresh from their dissection work in the morgue. He initiated the procedure of washing with a solution containing chlorine between all clinical activities. The results were extraordinary- the mortality rate from puerperal fever in the division fell from 18% in May 1847 to less than 3% in June–November of the same year [160,161,162].

Healthcare-associated pathogens have been recovered from frequently colonized areas of normal, intact patient skin, with the perineal or inguinal areas usually the most heavily colonized [164,165,166]. Approximately 10^6 skin squames containing viable microorganisms are shed daily from normal skin [167], therefore patient gowns, bed linen, bedside furniture, and other objects in the patient's immediate environment can easily become contaminated with patient flora [168,169]. Such contamination is likely to be caused by staphylococci or enterococci, which are resistant to dessication. It has been shown that organisms are transferred to various types of surfaces in much larger numbers from wet hands than from hands that are thoroughly dried [170]. Increased handwashing frequency among hospital staff has been associated with decreased transmission of infections among patients [171]. Hand hygiene includes handwashing with either plain or antiseptic-containing soap and water, and use of alcohol-based products that do not require the use of water (Table 1).

Besides hand-washing, the effectiveness of hand hygiene can be reduced by the type and length of fingernails [172]. In addition, the wearing of artificial nails has been shown to harbor more pathogenic organisms than natural nails [173]. It is recommended that artificial fingernails and extenders not be worn by healthcare personnel who have contact with high-risk patients due to the association with outbreaks of infections [174,175,176]. There is some evidence that jewelry affects the quality of hand hygiene; hand contamination with potential pathogens is increased with ring-wearing [177]. The Centers for Disease Control and Prevention (CDC) have issued recommendations and guideline for hand hygiene in health-care settings (Table 2).

Table 1. Antimicrobial Spectrum and Characteristics of Hand-Hygiene Antiseptic Agents* [163]

Group	Gram-positive bacteria	Gram-negative bacteria	Mycobacteria	Fungi	Viruses	Speed of action	Comments
Alcohols	+++	+++	+++	+++	+++	Fast	Optimum concentration 60%–95%; no persistent activity
Chlorhexidine (2%and 4% aqueous)	+++	++	+	+	+++	Intermediate	Persistent activity; rare allergic reactions
Iodine compounds	+++	+++	+++	++	+++	Intermediate	Causes skin burns; usually too irritating for hand hygiene
Iodophors	+++	+++	+	++	++	Intermediate	Less irritating than iodine; acceptance varies
Phenol derivatives	+++	+	+	+	+	Intermediate	Activity neutralized by nonionic surfactants
Tricolsan	+++	++	+	-	+++		
Quaternary ammonium compounds	+	++	—	—	+	Intermediate	Acceptability on hands varies
						Slow	Used only in combination with alcohols; ecologic concerns

Note: +++ = excellent; ++ = good, but does not include the entire bacterial spectrum; + = fair; — = no activity or not sufficient.

* Hexachlorophene is not included because it is no longer an accepted ingredient of hand disinfectants.

No recommendation were made regarding the routine use of non-alcohol-based hand rubs for hand hygiene in health-care settings, and the issue remains unresolved. In addition to the indications for hand-washing and hand antisepsis the CDC have also recommended hand-hygiene technique [163]. When decontaminating hands with an alcohol-based hand rub, apply product to palm of one hand and rub hands together, covering all surfaces of hands and fingers, until hands are dry. Follow the manufacturer's recommendations regarding the volume of product to use. When washing hands with soap and water, wet hands first with water, apply an amount of product recommended by the manufacturer to hands, and rub hands together vigorously for at least 15 seconds, covering all surfaces of the hands and fingers. Rinse hands with water and dry thoroughly with a disposable towel. Use towel to turn off the faucet. Avoid using hot water, because repeated exposure to hot water may increase the risk of dermatitis. Liquid, bar, leaflet or powdered forms of plain soap are acceptable when washing hands with a non-antimicrobial soap and water. When bar soap is used, soap racks that facilitate drainage and small bars of soap should be used. Multiple-use cloth towels of the hanging or roll type are not recommended for use in health-care settings. The hand-hygiene agents should be efficacious, and have low irritancy potential. The cost of hand-hygiene products should not be the primary factor influencing product selection. When selecting soaps or alcohol-based hand rubs, information from manufacturers should be elicited regarding any known interactions between products used to clean hands, skin care products, and the types of gloves used in the institution. Do not add soap to a partially empty soap dispenser as the practice of "topping off" dispensers can lead to bacterial contamination of soap.

Finally, there should be healthcare worker educational and motivational programs as part of an overall program to improve hand-hygiene practices, education of personnel regarding the types of patient-care activities that can result in hand contamination, and the advantages and disadvantages of various methods used to clean hands. There should be mechanisms in place to monitor workers adherence with recommended hand-hygiene practices and provide information regarding their performance.

Personal Protective Equipment (PPE)

Personal protective equipment refers to various barriers used alone or in combination to protect mucous membranes, airways, skin, and clothing from contact with infectious agents. The PPE used depends on the nature of the patient interaction and the likely mode of transmission. Special containers for used PPE should be placed at a convenient site to facilitate disposal and containment of contaminated materials. Hand hygiene is always the final step after removing and disposing of PPE.

Gloves are used to protect both patients and healthcare personnel from exposure to infectious material that may be carried on hands. They are used to prevent contamination of healthcare personnel hands when 1) anticipating direct contact with blood or body fluids, mucous membranes, broken skin and other potentially infectious material; 2) having direct contact with patients who are colonized or infected with pathogens transmitted by the contact route 3) handling or touching patient care equipment and potentially infected surfaces [174]. The selection of glove type use is based on the task that is to be performed, anticipated contact with chemicals and chemotherapeutic agents, latex sensitivity, sizing, and policies for a latex-free environment [178,179]. For contact with blood and body fluids during non-surgical patient care, a single pair of gloves generally provides adequate barrier protection [180]. During patient care, transmission of infectious organisms can be reduced by working from "clean" to "dirty" areas, and limiting contamination to surfaces that are directly needed for patient care. It may be necessary to change gloves during the care of a single patient to prevent cross-contamination of body sites [181]. Discarding gloves between patients is necessary to prevent transmission of infectious material. Gloves must not be washed for reuse because microorganisms cannot be totally removed from glove surfaces, and continued glove integrity cannot be ensured [182,183]. Gloves that fit snugly around the wrist are preferred for use with a gown because they cover the gown cuff and provide a continuous barrier for the forearms and hands. Glove puncture is fairly common, and the British Standard specification for surgical gloves accepts a 2% spontaneous leak rate [184]. Universal adoption of double-gloving is currently recommended in known high-risk situations, although double-gloving will not protect against penetrating sharps injuries. The significance, however, of unrecognized glove puncture from surgeon to patient is difficult to quantify. Hitherto it has been considered that macro-inoculation of tissues is virtually a prerequisite for seroconversion to occur as opposed to the very low level of contamination present on needles. For this to occur sufficient direct intravenous contamination of the blood must take place. It would now appear that micro-inoculation of tissue can also produce seroconversion [5].

Isolation gowns are used to protect the healthcare workers exposed body parts and to prevent contamination of clothing with blood, body fluids, and other potentially infectious material [185]. An isolation gown is worn if contact with blood or body fluid is anticipated, and in cases of contact with contaminated environmental surfaces. Full coverage of the arms and body front, from neck to the mid-thigh or below, ensures that clothing and exposed upper body areas are protected. Isolation gowns should be removed before leaving the patient environment to prevent possible contamination of areas outside the patient's room, and should be removed in a manner that prevents contamination of clothing or skin.

Masks are used for three purposes in healthcare settings: 1) to protect healthcare personnel from contact with infectious material from patients; 2) when engaged in sterile procedures to protect patients from exposure to infectious agents carried in a healthcare worker's mouth or nose, and 3) to limit dissemination of infectious respiratory secretions from the coughing patient to others. Masks with goggles or a face shield may be used to provide more complete protection for the face. Healthcare facilities need to stock different types of masks to meet individual healthcare personnel requirements.

Goggles, in addition to a mask, aids in preventing exposure to infectious agents transmitted via respiratory droplets. While effective as eye protection, goggles do not provide splash or spray protection to other parts of the face. It is important to remember that even if droplet precautions are not recommended for a specific pathogen, protection for the eyes, nose and mouth by using a mask and goggles or a face shield is necessary when it is likely that there will be a splash or spray of respiratory secretions or other body fluids. Disposable or non-disposable face shields may be used as an alternative to goggles [186]. As compared with goggles, a face shield can provide protection to other facial areas in addition to the eyes. Personal eyeglasses and contact lenses are not considered adequate eye protection [186].

Aerosol-generating procedures, such as bronchoscopy, endotracheal intubation, and open suctioning of the respiratory tract, have been associated with transmission of infections to healthcare personnel [46,187]. Protection of the eyes, nose and mouth, in addition to gown and gloves, is recommended during performance of these procedures. Use of a particulate respirator is recommended during aerosol-generating procedures. In areas where the need for resuscitation is unpredictable, mouthpieces, pocket resuscitation masks with one-way valves, and other ventilation devices provide an alternative to mouth-to-mouth resuscitation, preventing exposure of the caregiver's nose and mouth to oral and respiratory fluids during the procedure.

Surgical Attire

Surgical attire refers to scrub suits, caps/hoods, shoe covers, masks, gloves, and gowns.

Sterile surgical gowns and drapes are used to create a barrier between the surgical field and potential sources of infection. Gowns are worn by all scrubbed surgical team members and drapes are placed over the patient. Gowns and drapes are classified as disposable for single use or reusable. Regardless of the material used to manufacture gowns and drapes, these items should be impermeable to liquids and viruses [188,189].

Table 2. Recommendations and Guideline for Hand Hygiene in Health-Care Settings Modified from [163 Centers for Disease Control and Prevention. Guideline for Hand Hygiene in Health-Care Settings: Recommendations of the Healthcare Infection Control Practices Advisory Committee and the HICPAC/SHEA/APIC/IDSA Hand Hygiene Task Force. MMWR 2002;51(No. RR- 16)].

Indications for handwashing and hand antisepsis	Condition	Action
	Hands visibly dirty or contaminated with proteinaceous material or visibly soiled with blood or other body fluids	Wash hands with either a non-antimicrobial soap and water, or an antimicrobial soap and water
	Hands are not visibly soiled - in all clinical situations	Use an alcohol-based hand rub or wash hands with an antimicrobial soap and water
	Before direct contact with patients, before donning sterile gloves when inserting a central intravascular catheter, before inserting indwelling urinary catheters, peripheral vascular catheters, or other invasive devices, before eating and after using a restroom After contact with a patient's intact skin (e.g., when taking a pulse or blood pressure, and lifting a patient), after contact with body fluids or excretions, mucous membranes, nonintact skin, and wound dressings, contact with inanimate objects in the immediate vicinity of the patient, after removing gloves, When moving from a contaminated-body site to a clean-body site during patient care. If exposure to *Bacillus anthracis* is suspected or proven	Decontaminate hands

Table 2. (Continued)

Surgical hand antisepsis	Condition	Action
	Before beginning surgical hand scrub	Remove rings, watches, and bracelets Remove debris from underneath fingernails using a nail cleaner under running water
	Before donning sterile gloves when performing surgical procedures	Surgical hand antisepsis using an antimicrobial soap or alcohol-based hand rub with persistent activity
	Before applying the alcohol solution	Prewash hands and forearms with non-antimicrobial soap and dry hands and forearms completely
	After application of the alcohol-based product	Allow hands and forearms to dry thoroughly before donning sterile gloves
Other Aspects of Hand Hygiene	**Condition**	**Action**
	Direct contact with patients at high risk (e.g., in ICU or operating rooms	Do not wear artificial fingernails or extenders Keep natural nails tips less than 1/4-inch long
	Contact with blood or other potentially infectious materials, mucous membranes, and nonintact skin	Wear gloves
	After caring for a patient	Remove gloves Do not wear the same pair of gloves for the care of more than one patient Do not wash gloves between uses with different patients
	During patient care if moving from a contaminated body site to a clean body site	Change gloves

Administrative measures	Condition	Action
	Hand-hygiene adherence	Prioritize Provide appropriate administrative support Provide appropriate financial resources
	Adherence to recommended hand-hygiene practices	Implement multidisciplinary program
	Improve hand-hygiene adherence	Provide HCWs with accessible alcohol-based hand-rub product Make alcohol-based hand rub available at entrance to the patient's room, at the bedside, in other convenient locations

Experimental data has shown that live microorganisms are shed from hair, exposed skin, and mucous membranes of operating room personnel, therefore the use of barriers seems prudent to minimize a patient's exposure to the skin, mucous membranes, or hair of surgical team members, as well as to protect surgical team members from exposure to blood and bloodborne pathogens [190,191,192]. Surgical caps/hoods are inexpensive and reduce contamination of the surgical field by organisms isolated from the hair or scalp. Surgical-site infection outbreaks have occasionally been traced to organisms isolated even when caps were worn by personnel during the operation and in the operating suites [190,193]. The use of shoe covers has not been shown to decrease surgical-site infection risk or to decrease bacterial counts on the operating room floor [194,195]. Shoe covers may, however, protect surgical team members from exposure to blood and other body fluids during an operation. For operative delivery and other surgical procedures where blood spillage is common, the use of waterproof gowns, surgical caps and wellington boots is recommended. In high-risk situations, over-shoes should be worn over the boots as these can be discarded at the edge of the contaminated area thereby eliminating the walking of blood and contamination outside the surgical area. Boots are necessary for personal protection in the gap below the protective apron [5].

Prevention of Needlestick and Other Sharps-Related Injuries

Transmission of hepatitis B, hepatitis C and HIV to healthcare personnel have been reported due to needle injuries and other sharps [196]. The prevention of sharps injuries include measures to handle needles and other sharp devices, and dispose of them appropriately such that there is no injury to the user or others who may encounter the device during or after a procedure. CDC has provided guidance on sharps injury prevention [197]. In essence they focus on the appropriate design and convenient placement of puncture-resistant sharps disposal containers and the education of healthcare personnel on the dangers of recapping, bending, and breaking used needles. Other strategies include the use of alternate routes for medication delivery and vaccination when available, reviewing specimen collection systems to identify opportunities to eliminate unnecessary punctures, simple obvious technique at surgery, using instruments rather than fingers to grasp needles, retract tissue, and load/unload needles and scalpels, give verbal warnings when passing sharps, avoiding hand-to-hand passage of sharp instruments by using a basin or neutral zone, using alternative cutting methods such as blunt electrocautery and laser devices when appropriate, substituting endoscopic surgery for open surgery when possible; and using round-tipped scalpel blades instead of sharp-tipped blades. Additional recommendations are the education of staff in reducing the use of invasive procedures, an adequate staff-to-patient ratio, formation of a needlestick prevention committee for compulsory in-service education programs, out-sourcing of replacement and disposal of sharps boxes, and the adoption and evaluation of a needle-less intravenous access system, safety syringes, and a pre-filled cartridge needle-less system.

An important aspect of prevention of infectivity is the adoption of universal body fluid precautions in clinical practice. The CDC has issued guidance recommending the adoption of universal body fluid precautions in clinical practice [68]. The objectives must be:

1. An understanding of the routes of transmission and infectivity of HIV and hepatitis B.
2. A non-judgemental approach to those who are or may be seropositive.
3. Meticulous observance of high standards of clinical hygiene in all circumstances, ie. Standard Precautions.
4. Managerial responsibility for provision of protective clothing and decontamination.
5. Application of these principles to major surgery of all forms.

Management of Penetrating Injuries [5]

Any penetrating injury of a surgeon or assistant during a surgical procedure should raise consideration of the possibility of viral transmission. The first immediate action must be to irrigate the wound with copious fresh water without scrubbing. Bleeding should be encouraged. Thereafter, other relevant steps need to be taken.

1. The sero-status of the patient undergoing the surgical procedure: if this has not been determined before operation it may be possible for the patient to give consent for a test without being told the result. This would avoid the problems of non-disclosure to individuals.
2. Storage of a serum sample taken from the injured operator: it may be prudent to have a serum sample stored (but not necessarily tested) for future reference if required.
3. Occupational health advice is necessary if the patient concerned is in a high-risk group or is known to be HIV positive. Counseling may well be required and serial tests over a period of months be advised. The question of post-exposure prophylaxis

will be raised in such cases. Ideally such prophylaxis should be instituted within an hour of contamination injury.

4. If the injury has occurred from a known HIV-positive source the operator, if commonly engaged in invasive surgical practice, will need to seek professional advice as to the propriety of continuing to work during the potential 'window' period before seroconversion.

Patient Placement

Hospital patient placement includes single patient rooms, two patient rooms, and multi-bed wards. Of these, single patient rooms are preferred when there is concern about transmission of an infectious agent [198]. In the absence of infectious diseases that require isolation rooms, the risk of transmission of infectious agents is not considered when making placement decisions. When there are a limited number of single-patient rooms, it is best to prioritize them for those patients who have conditions that facilitate transmission of infectious material to other patients, and for those who are at increased risk of acquiring the transmitted infections [199]. During an outbreak caused by a gastrointestinal tract pathogen, use of single patient rooms with a private bathroom limits transmission, especially when the colonized or infected patient has poor personal hygiene, fecal incontinence, or cannot be expected to implement procedures that prevent transmission of microorganisms. In the absence of continued transmission, it is not necessary to provide a private bathroom for patients colonized or infected with enteric pathogens as long as personal hygiene practices and Standard Precautions, especially hand hygiene, and appropriate environmental cleaning are maintained [68]. The assignment of a dedicated commode to a patient, and cleaning and disinfecting fixtures and equipment that may be contaminated are especially important when a single-patient room can not be used [200]. Studies have shown that being in the same room with a colonized or infected patient is not necessarily a risk factor for transmission, however, for children the risk of transmissible diarrhea is increased with the increased number of patients per room [201,202].

Cohorting is the practice of grouping together patients who are colonized or infected with the same organism to confine their care to one area and prevent contact with other patients. Cohorts are created based on clinical diagnosis, microbiologic confirmation, epidemiology, and mode of transmission of the infectious agent. Cohorting is often implemented after routine infection control measures have failed to control an outbreak. Cohorting healthcare personnel to care only for patients infected or colonized with a single target pathogen limits further transmission of the pathogen to uninfected patients [203].

Patients actively infected with or incubating transmissible infectious diseases are often encountered in ambulatory settings; healthcare workers in outpatient settings should implement source containment measures such as asking coughing patients to wear a surgical mask to prevent transmission of respiratory infections. Signs can be posted at the entrance to facilities or at the reception desk requesting that the patient, or individuals accompanying the patient, inform the receptionist if there are symptoms of a respiratory infection, gastroenteritis, skin rash, or exposure to a transmissible disease. Placement of potentially infectious patients without delay in an examination room away from the common waiting area limits the number of exposed individuals to potentially infectious agents [204].

Environmental Measures

Cleaning and disinfecting surfaces in patient-care areas are part of Standard Precautions. The cleaning and disinfection of patient-care areas is important for frequently touched surfaces that are most likely to be contaminated [205]. The frequency of cleaning needs to change based on the patient's level of hygiene and the degree of environmental contamination. During a suspected or proven outbreak where an environmental reservoir is suspected, routine cleaning procedures should be reviewed, and the need for additional trained cleaning staff should be assessed. Disinfectants and detergents that best meet the overall needs of the healthcare facility for routine cleaning and disinfection should be selected [206]. The need to change disinfectants based on the presence of more resistant organisms can be determined in consultation with the infection control committee [207].

Patient care Equipment and Instruments/Devices

Medical equipment must be cleaned and maintained according to the manufacturers' instructions to prevent patient-to-patient transmission of infectious agents [208]. Cleaning and removal of organic material should always precede disinfection and sterilization of instruments and devices because residual organic material may reduce the efficacy of the disinfection and sterilization processes [206]. Equipment, such as commodes, intravenous pumps, and ventilators, should be thoroughly cleaned and disinfected before use on another patient. It is important to include computers and personal digital assistants used in patient care in policies for cleaning and disinfection as reports have linked computer contamination to colonization and infections in patients [209].

Visitors to healthcare facilities may be the source of several types of acquired infections. Visitor screening is especially important during community outbreaks of infectious diseases and for high risk patient units. Screening of visitors before they are allowed into clinical areas is necessary to prevent the introduction of illnesses, especially common respiratory infections. Screening may be passive through the use of signs to alert visitors with signs and symptoms of communicable diseases not to enter clinical areas, or more active screening such as the completion of a questionnaire related to recent exposures or current symptoms. If exclusion is not considered appropriate, then the symptomatic visitor must wear a mask while in the healthcare facility and remain in the patient's room thereby avoiding exposure to others.

Important adjunctive measures that are not considered primary components of programs to prevent transmission of infectious agents but improve the effectiveness of such programs, include 1) antimicrobial management programs; 2) postexposure chemoprophylaxis with antiviral or antibacterial agents; 3) vaccines used both for pre and postexposure prevention [68]. Certain immunizations, such as hepatitis B, rubella, influenza, and varicella vaccines, recommended for susceptible healthcare personnel have decreased the risk of infection and the potential for transmission in healthcare facilities [210,211,212].

Conclusion

Infection control is an essential component of care and one which has too often been undervalued in recent years. Control of infection depends upon identifying the mode of spread and interrupting the chain of infection, its replication and spread. Infection-control strategies and engineering controls, when consistently implemented, are effective in preventing opportunistic environmentally-related infections. Standard Precautions are designed to improve the level of protection afforded to patients and staff within the healthcare environment. Adherence to Standard Precautions, proper use of disinfectants, proper maintenance of medical equipment, water-quality standards, proper ventilation standards for specialized care environments, and protective wear will minimize health-care-associated infection risks and reduce the frequency of pseudo-outbreaks. Studies have shown that a good infection control program can reduce infection rates by 32% [132]. The importance of a high level safe clinical practice cannot be overestimated.

References

[1] Kohn, LT; Corrigan, JM; Donaldson, MS. (eds.) In: *To Err Is Human: Building a Safer Health System*, Washington, DC: National Academy Press; 2000

[2] Guidelines for environmental infection control in health-care facilities. Recommendations of CDC and the Healthcare Infection Control Practices Advisory Committee. 2003. Available from: www.cdc.gov/ncidod/hip/enviro/guide.htm. Accessed on 27 July 2008

[3] Good practice in infection prevention and control. Guidance for nursing staff 2005. Available from http://www.rcn.org.uk/__data/assets/pdf_file/0003/78654/002741.pdf. Accessed on 25 August 2008

[4] Bennett, JV. Brachman, PS. (eds.) *The inanimate environment*, In: Rhame FS. Hospital Infections, 4th ed. Philadelphia, PA: Lippincott-Raven, 1998, 299–324

[5] Hudson, CN. Nosocomial infection and infection control Procedure. *Baillieres Clin Obstet Gynaecol 1992*, *6(1)*, 137-148

[6] Welch, J; Webster, M; Tilzey, AJ; et al. Hepatitis-B infections after gynaecological surgery. *Lancet* 1989, i: 205-207

[7] European Collaborative Study. Children born to women with HIV-1 infection: natural history and risk of transmission. *Lancet*, 1991, 337, 253-260

[8] Marcus, R. The Co-operative Needlestick Surveillance Group: Surveillance of health care workers exposed to blood from patients infected with the human immunodeficiency virus. *N Eng J Med*, 1988, 319, 1118-1123

[9] Henderson, DK; Fahey, BJ; Willy, M; et al. Risk for occupational transmission of human immunodeficiency virus type I, associated with clinical exposure. *Ann Intern Med*, 1990, 113, 740-746

[10] Morbidity and Mortality Weekly Report Centre for Disease Control. Possible transmission of human immunodeficiency virus to a patient during an invasive dental procedure. *MMWR*, 1990, 39, 29

[11] Osterholm, M; Hedberg, C. *Epidemiology of infectious diseases*, In: Mandell G, Bennett J, Dolin R., (eds.). Philadelphia, PA: Churchill Livingstone; 2005. pp. 161–173

[12] Thomsen, RW; Hundborg, HH; Lervang, HH; et al. Risk of community-acquired pneumococcal bacteremia in patients with diabetes: a population-based case-control study. *Diabetes Care*, 2004, 27(5), 1143-1147

[13] Carton, JA; Maradona, JA; Nuno, FJ; et al. Diabetes mellitus and bacteraemia: a comparative study between diabetic and non-diabetic patients. *Eur J Med*, 1992, 1(5), 281-287

[14] Hirschtick, RE; Glassroth, J; Jordan, MC; et al. Bacterial pneumonia in persons infected with the human immunodeficiency virus. Pulmonary Complications of HIV Infection Study Group. *N Engl J Med*, 1995, 333(13), 845-851

[15] Rosenberg, AL; Seneff, MG; Atiyeh L; et al. The importance of bacterial sepsis in intensive care unit patients with acquired immunodeficiency syndrome: implications for future care in the age of increasing antiretroviral resistance. *Crit Care Med*, 2001, 29(3), 548-556

[16] Malone, JL; Ijaz, K; Lambert, L; et al. Investigation of healthcare-associated transmission of Mycobacterium tuberculosis among patients with malignancies at three hospitals and at a residential facility. *Cancer*, 2004, 101(12), 2713-2721

[17] Fishman, JA; Rubin, RH. Infection in organ-transplant recipients. *N Engl J Med* 1998;338(24), 1741-1751

[18] Safdar, N; Kluger, DM; Maki, DG. A review of risk factors for catheterrelated bloodstream infection caused by percutaneously inserted, noncuffed central venous catheters: implications for preventive strategies. *Medicine*, (Baltimore) 2002, 81(6), 466-479

[19] Yogaraj, JS; Elward, AM; Fraser VJ. Rate, risk factors, and outcomes of nosocomial primary bloodstream infection in pediatric intensive care unit patients. *Pediatrics*, 2002, 110(3), 481-485

[20] Donlan, RM. Biofilms: microbial life on surfaces. *Emerg Infect Dis*, 2002, 8(9), 881-890

[21] Bonten, MJ; Slaughter, S; Hayden, MK; et al. External sources of vancomycin-resistant enterococci for intensive care units. *Crit Care Med*, 1998, 26(12), 2001-2004

[22] Flynn, DM; Weinstein, RA; Nathan, C; et al. Patients' endogenous flora as the source of "nosocomial" Enterobacter in cardiac surgery. *J Infect Dis*, 1987, 156(2), 363-8

[23] Olson, B; Weinstein, RA; Nathan, C; et al. Epidemiology of endemic Pseudomonas aeruginosa: why infection control efforts have failed. *J Infect Dis*, 1984, 150(6), 808-816

[24] Perl, TM; Cullen, JJ; Wenzel, RP; et al. Intranasal mupirocin to prevent postoperative Staphylococcus aureus infections. *N Engl J Med*, 2002, 346(24), 1871-1877

[25] Toltzis, P; Hoyen, C; Spinner-Block, S; et al. Factors that predict preexisting colonization with antibiotic-resistant gram-negative bacilli in patients admitted to a pediatric intensive care unit. *Pediatrics*, 1999, 103 (4 Pt1):719-723

[26] Rosen, H.R. Acquisition of hepatitis C by a conjunctival splash. *Am J Infect Control*, 1997, 25(3), 242-247

[27] Beltrami, EM; Kozak, A; Williams, IT; et al. Transmission of HIV and hepatitis C virus from a nursing home patient to a health care worker. *Am J Infect Control*, 2003, 31(3), 168-175

[28] Obasanjo, OO; Wu, P; Conlon, M; et al. An outbreak of scabies in a teaching hospital: lessons learned. *Infect Control Hosp Epidemiol*, 2001, 22(1), 13-8

[29] Andersen, BM; Haugen, H; Rasch, M; et al. Outbreak of scabies in Norwegian nursing homes and home care patients: control and prevention. *J Hosp Infect*, 2000, 45(2), 160-164

[30] Avitzur, Y; Amir, J; Herpetic whitlow infection in a general pediatrician-an occupational hazard. *Infection*, 2002, 30(4), 234-236

[31] Adams, G; Stover BH; Keenlyside, RA; et al. Nosocomial herpetic infections in a pediatric intensive care unit. *Am J Epidemiol*, 1981, 113(2), 126-132

[32] Boyce, JM; Pittet, D. Guideline for Hand Hygiene in Health-Care Settings. Recommendations of the Healthcare Infection Control Practices Advisory Committee and the HICPAC/SHEA/APIC/IDSA Hand Hygiene Task Force. Society for Healthcare Epidemiology of America/Association for Professionals in Infection Control/Infectious Diseases Society of America. *MMWR Recomm Rep*, 2002, 51(RR-16), 1-45

[33] Bhalla, A; Pultz, NJ; Gries, DM; et al. Acquisition of nosocomial pathogens on hands after contact with environmental surfaces near hospitalized patients. *Infect Control Hosp Epidemiol*, 2004, 25(2), 164-167

[34] Duckro, AN; Blom, DW; Lyle, EA; et al. Transfer of vancomycin-resistant enterococci via health care worker hands. *Arch Intern Med*, 2005, 165(3), 302-307

[35] Desenclos, JC; Bourdiol-Razes, M; Rolin, B; et al. Hepatitis C in a ward for cystic fibrosis and diabetic patients: possible transmission by springloaded finger-stick devices for self-monitoring of capillary blood glucose. *Infect Control Hosp Epidemiol*, 2001, 22(11), 701-707

[36] Brooks, SE; Veal, RO; Kramer, M; et al. Reduction in the incidence of Clostridium difficile-associated diarrhea in an acute care hospital and a skilled nursing facility following replacement of electronic thermometers with single-use disposables. *Infect Control Hosp Epidemiol*, 1992, 13(2), 98-103

[37] Hall, CB; Douglas, RG. Jr. Modes of transmission of respiratory syncytial virus. *J Pediatr*, 1981, 99(1), 100-103

[38] Buttery, JP; Alabaster, SJ; Heine, RG; et al. Multiresistant Pseudomonas aeruginosa outbreak in a pediatric oncology ward related to bath toys. *Pediatr Infect Dis J*, 1998, 17(6), 509-513

[39] Bronowicki, JP; Venard, V; Botte, C; et al. Patient-to-patient transmission of hepatitis C virus during colonoscopy. *N Engl J Med*, 1997, 337(4), 237-240

[40] Michele, TM; Cronin, WA; Graham, NM; et al. Transmission of Mycobacterium tuberculosis by a fiberoptic bronchoscope. Identification by DNA fingerprinting. *JAMA*, 1997, 278(13), 1093-1095

[41] Weber, DJ; Rutala, WA. Lessons from outbreaks associated with bronchoscopy. *Infect Control Hosp Epidemiol*, 2001, 22(7), 403-408

[42] Zachary, KC; Bayne, PS; Morrison, VJ; et al. Contamination of gowns, gloves, and stethoscopes with vancomycinresistant enterococci. *Infect Control Hosp Epidemiol*, 2001, 22(9), 560-564

[43] Perry, C; Marshall, R; Jones, E. Bacterial contamination of uniforms. *J Hosp Infect*, 2001, 48(3), 238-241

[44] Papineni, R.S. & Rosenthal, F.S. The size distribution of droplets in the exhaled breath of healthy human subjects. *J Aerosol Med*, 1997, 10(2), 105-116

[45] Wells, WF. On airborne infection: Study II. Droplets and droplet nuclei. *Am J Hygiene*, 1934, 20, 611-618

[46] Fowler, RA; Guest, CB; Lapinsky, SE; et al. Transmission of severe acute respiratory syndrome during intubation and mechanical ventilation. *Am J Respir Crit Care Med*, 2004, 169(11), 1198-1202

[47] Ensor, E; Humphreys, H; Peckham, D; et al. Is Burkholderia (Pseudomonas) cepacia disseminated from cystic fibrosis patients during physiotherapy? *J Hosp Infect*, 1996, 32(1), 9-15

[48] Christian, MD; Loutfy, M; McDonald, LC; et al. Possible SARS coronavirus transmission during cardiopulmonary resuscitation. *Emerg Infect Dis*, 2004, 10(2), 287-293

[49] Valenzuela, TD; Hooton, TM; Kaplan, EL; et al. Transmission of 'toxic strep' syndrome from an infected child to a firefighter during CPR. *Ann Emerg Med*, 1991, 20(1), 90-92

[50] Hall, CB; Douglas, RG, Jr; Schnabel, KC; et al. Infectivity of respiratory syncytial virus by various routes of inoculation. *Infect Immun*, 1981, 33(3), 779-783

[51] Feigin, RD; Baker, CJ; Herwaldt, LA; et al. Epidemic meningococcal disease in an elementary-school classroom. *N Engl J Med*, 1982, 307(20), 1255-1257

[52] Dick, EC; Jennings, LC; Mink, KA; et al. Aerosol transmission of rhinovirus colds. *J Infect Dis*, 1987, 156(3), 442-448

[53] Duguid, JP. The size and duration of air-carriage of respiratory droplets and droplet nucleii. *J Hyg*, (Lond) 1946, 44, 471-479

[54] Cole, EC; Cook, CE. Characterization of infectious aerosols in health care facilities: an aid to effective engineering controls and preventive strategies. *Am J Infect Control*, 1998, 26(4), 453-464

[55] Bloch, AB; Orenstein, WA; Ewing, WM; et al. Measles outbreak in a pediatric practice: airborne transmission in an office setting. *Pediatrics* 1985, 75(4), 676-683

[56] LeClair, JM; Zaia, JA; Levin, MJ; et al. Airborne transmission of chickenpox in a hospital. *N Engl J Med*, 1980, 302(8), 450-453

[57] Riley, RL; Mills, CC; Nyka, W; et al. Aerial dissemination of pulmonary tuberculosis. A two-year study of contagion in a tuberculosis ward. 1959. *Am J Hyg*, 1959, 70, 185-196

[58] Moser, MR; Bender, TR; Margolis, HS; et al. An outbreak of influenza aboard a commercial airliner. *Am J Epidemiol*, 1979, 110(1), 1-6

[59] Alford, RH; Kasel, JA; Gerone, PJ; et al. Human influenza resulting from aerosol inhalation. *Proc Soc Exp Biol Med*, 1966, 122(3), 800-804

[60] Chadwick, PR; McCann, R. Transmission of a small round structured virus by vomiting during a hospital outbreak of gastroenteritis. *J Hosp Infect*, 1994, 26(4), 251-259

[61] Prince, DS; Astry, C; Vonderfecht, S; et al. Aerosol transmission of experimental rotavirus infection. *Pediatr Infect Dis*, 1986, 5(2), 218-222

[62] Sawyer, LA; Murphy, JJ; Kaplan, JE; et al. 25- to 30-nm virus particle associated with a hospital outbreak of acute gastroenteritis with evidence for airborne transmission. *Am J Epidemiol*, 1988, 127(6), 1261-1271

[63] Marks, PJ; Vipond, IB; Carlisle, D; et al. Evidence for airborne transmission of Norwalk-like virus (NLV) in a hotel restaurant. *Epidemiol Infect*, 2000, 124(3), 481-487

[64] Dull, PM; Wilson, KE; Kournikakis, B; et al. Bacillus anthracis aerosolization associated with a contaminated mail sorting machine. *Emerg Infect Dis*, 2002, 8(10), 1044-1047

[65] Weis, CP; Intrepido, AJ; Miller, AK; et al. Secondary aerosolization of viable Bacillus anthracis spores in a contaminated US Senate Office. *JAMA*, 2002, 288(22), 2853-2858

[66] Patterson, JE; Zidouh, A; Miniter, P; et al. Hospital epidemiologic surveillance for invasive aspergillosis: patient demographics and the utility of antigen detection. *Infect Control Hosp Epidemiol*, 1997, 18(2), 104-108

[67] Arnow, PM; Andersen, RL; Mainous, PD; et al. Pumonary aspergillosis during hospital renovation. *Am Rev Respir Dis*, 1978, 118(1), 49-53

[68] Siegel, JD; Rhinehart, E; Jackson, M; et al, and the Healthcare Infection Control Practices Advisory Committee. Guideline for Isolation Precautions: Preventing Transmission of Infectious Agents in Healthcare Settings 2007. Available at *http://www.cdc.gov/ncidod/dhqp/pdf/isolation*, 2007. *pdf* Accessed on 10 August 2008

[69] Nguyen, GT; Proctor, SE; Sinkowitz-Cochran, RL; et al. Status of infection surveillance and control programs in the United States, 1992-1996. Association for Professionals in Infection Control and Epidemiology, Inc. *Am J Infect Control*, 2000, 28(6), 392-400

[70] Richards, C; Emori, TG; Edwards, J; et al. Characteristics of hospitals and infection control professionals participating in the National Nosocomial Infections Surveillance System 1999. *Am J Infect Control*, 2001, 29(6), 400-403

[71] Srinivasan, A; McDonald, LC; Jernigan, D; et al. Foundations of the severe acute respiratory syndrome preparedness and response plan for healthcare facilities. *Infect Control Hosp Epidemiol*, 2004, 25(12), 1020-1025

[72] CDC. Guidelines for preventing the transmission of Mycobacterium tuberculosis in health-care settings. *MMWR Recomm Rep*, 2005, 54(17), 1-141

[73] Wenzel, RP; Thompson, RL; Landry, SM; et al. Hospital-acquired infections in intensive care unit patients: an overview with emphasis on epidemics. *Infect Control*, 1983, 4(5), 371-375

[74] Wenzel, RP; Gennings, C. Bloodstream infections due to Candida species in the intensive care unit: identifying especially high-risk patients to determine prevention strategies. *Clin Infect Dis*, 2005, 41 Suppl 6, S389-393

[75] San Miguel, LG; Cobo, J; Otheo, E; et al. Secular trends of candidemia in a large tertiary-care hospital from 1988 to 2000. emergence of Candida parapsilosis. *Infect Control Hosp Epidemiol*, 2005, 26(6), 548-552

[76] NNIS. National Nosocomial Infections Surveillance (NNIS) System Report, data summary from January 1992 through June 2004. *Am J Infect Control*, 2004, 32(8), 470-485

[77] Husni, RN; Goldstein, LS; Arroliga, AC; et al. Risk factors for an outbreak of multi-drug-resistant Acinetobacter nosocomial pneumonia among intubated patients. *Chest*, 1999, 115(5), 1378-1382

[78] McDonald, LC; Walker, M; Carson, L; et al. Outbreak of Acinetobacter spp. bloodstream infections in a nursery associated with contaminated aerosols and air conditioners. *Pediatr Infect Dis J*, 1998, 17(8), 716-722

[79] Trick, WE; Kioski, CM; Howard, KM; et al. Outbreak of Pseudomonas aeruginosa ventriculitis among patients in a neurosurgical intensive care unit. *Infect Control Hosp Epidemiol*, 2000, 21(3), 204-208

[80] Pruitt, BA, Jr; McManus, AT; Kim, SH; et al. Burn wound infections: current status. *World J Surg*, 1998, 22(2), 135-145

[81] Weber, J. (ed). Epidemiology of Infections and Strategies for Control in Burn Care and Therapy. St. Louis: Mosby, Inc.; 1998

[82] Heggers, JP; McCoy, L; Reisner, B; et al. Alternate antimicrobial therapy for vancomycin-resistant enterococci burn wound infections. *J Burn Care Rehabil*, 1998, 19(5), 399-403

[83] Sheridan, RL; Weber, J; Benjamin, J; et al. Control of methicillin-resistant Staphylococcus aureus in a pediatric burn unit. *Am J Infect Control*, 1994, 22(6), 340-345

[84] McGregor, JC. Profile of the first four years of the Regional Burn Unit based at St. John's Hospital, West Lothian (1992-1996). *J R Coll Surg Edinb*, 1998, 43(1), 45-48

[85] Desai, MH; Rutan, RL; Heggers, JP; et al. Candida infection with and without nystatin prophylaxis. A 11-year experience with patients with burn injury. *Arch Surg*, 1992, 127(2), 159-162

[86] Bowser-Wallace, BH; Graves, DB; Caldwell, FT. An epidemiological profile and trend analysis of wound flora in burned children: 7 years' experience. *Burns Incl Therm Inj*, 1984, 11(1), 16-25

[87] Meier, PA; Carter, CD; Wallace, SE; et al. A prolonged outbreak of methicillin-resistant Staphylococcus aureus in the burn unit of a tertiary medical center. *Infect Control Hosp Epidemiol*, 1996, 17(12), 798-802

[88] Lee JJ; Marvin JA; Heimbach DM, Grube BJ, Engrav LH. Infection control in a burn center. J Burn Care Rehabil 1990, 11(6), 575-580

[89] Moster, D; Lie, RT; Markestad, T. Long-term medical and social consequences of preterm birth. *N Eng J Med*, 2008, 359, 262-273

[90] Raymond, J; Aujard, Y. Nosocomial infections in pediatric patients: a European, multicenter prospective study. European Study Group. *Infect Control Hosp Epidemiol*, 2000, 21(4), 260-263

[91] Allen, U; Ford-Jones, EL. Nosocomial infections in the pediatric patient: an update. *Am J Infect Control*, 1990, 18(3), 176-193

[92] Grohskopf, LA; Sinkowitz-Cochran, RL; Garrett, DO; et al. A national point-prevalence survey of pediatric intensive care unit-acquired infections in the United States. *J Pediatr*, 2002, 140(4), 432-438

[93] Sohn, AH; Garrett, DO; Sinkowitz-Cochran, RL; et al. Prevalence of nosocomial infections in neonatal intensive care unit patients: Resultsfrom the first national point-prevalence survey. *J Pediatr*, 2001, 139(6), 821-827

[94] Gaynes, RP; Edwards, JR; Jarvis, WR; et al. Nosocomial infections among neonates in high-risk nurseries in the United States. National Nosocomial Infections Surveillance System. *Pediatrics* 1996, 98(3 Pt 1), 357-361

[95] Avila-Aguero, ML; German, G; Paris, MM; et al. Toys in a pediatric hospital: are they a bacterial source? *Am J Infect Control*, 2004, 32(5), 287-290

[96] Jarvis, WR; Robles, B. Nosocomial infections in pediatric patients. *Adv Pediatr Infect Dis*, 1996, 12:243-295

[97] Jarvis, WR. Infection control and changing health-care delivery systems. *Emerg Infect Dis*, 2001, 7(2), 170-173
[98] White, MC. Identifying infectious diseases in prisons: surveillance, protection, and intervention. *West J Med*, 1999, 170(3), 177
[99] Puisis, M. Update on public health in correctional facilities. *West J Med*, 1998, 169(6), 374
[100] CDC. Tuberculosis transmission in a homeless shelter population—New York, 2000-2003. *MMWR Morb Mortal Wkly Rep*, 2005, 54(6), 149-152
[101] Parece, MS; Herrera, GA; Voigt, RF; et al. STD testing policies and practices in U.S. city and county jails. *Sex Transm Dis*, 1999, 26(8), 431-437
[102] CDC. Prevention and Control of Tuberculosis in Correctional Facilities. Recommendations of the Advisory Council for the Elimination of Tuberculosis. *MMWR Recomm Rep*, 1996, 45(RR-8), 1-37
[103] Stevenson, K.B. Regional data set of infection rates for long-term care facilities: description of a valuable benchmarking tool. *Am J Infect Control*, 1999, 27(1), 20-26
[104] Jackson, MM ; Fierer, J ; Barrett-Connor, E ; et al. Intensive surveillance for infections in a three-year study of nursing home patients. *Am J Epidemiol*, 1992, 135(6), 685-696
[105] Perls, TT. Herget, M. Higher respiratory infection rates on an Alzheimer's special care unit and successful intervention. *J Am Geriatr Soc*, 1995, 43(12), 1341-1344
[106] Richards, CL. Infections in Long-Term-Care Facilities: Screen or Clean? *Infect Control Hosp Epidemiol*, 2005, 26(10), 800-801
[107] Loeb, MB; Craven, S; McGeer, AJ; et al. Risk factors for resistance to antimicrobial agents among nursing home residents. *Am J Epidemiol*, 2003, 157(1), 40-47
[108] Allard, JP; Aghdassi, E; McArthur, M; et al. Nutrition risk factors for survival in the elderly living in Canadian long-term care facilities. *J Am Geriatr Soc*, 2004, 52(1), 59-65
[109] Pick, N; McDonald, A; Bennett, N; et al. Pulmonary aspiration in a longterm care setting: clinical and laboratory observations and an analysis of risk factors. *J Am Geriatr Soc*, 1996, 44(7), 763-768
[110] Nicolle, L.E. The chronic indwelling catheter and urinary infection in longterm- care facility residents. *Infect Control Hosp Epidemiol*, 2001, 22(5), 316-321
[111] Pien, EC; Hume, KE; Pien, FD. Gastrostomy tube infections in a community hospital. *Am J Infect Control*, 1996, 24(5), 353-358
[112] Bula, CJ; Ghilardi, G, Wietlisbach, V; et al. Infections and functional impairment in nursing home residents: a reciprocal relationship. *J Am Geriatr Soc*, 2004, 52(5), 700-706
[113] Trick, WE; Weinstein, RA; DeMarais, PL; et al. Colonization of skilled-care facility residents with antimicrobial-resistant pathogens. *J Am Geriatr Soc*, 2001, 49(3), 270-276
[114] Mylotte, JM; Goodnough, S; Tayara, A. Antibiotic-resistant organisms among long-term care facility residents on admission to an inpatient geriatrics unit: Retrospective and prospective surveillance. *Am J Infect Control*, 2001, 29(3), 139-144
[115] Pop-Vicas, AE. D'Agata, E.M. The rising influx of multidrug-resistant gram-negative bacilli into a tertiary care hospital. *Clin Infect Dis*, 2005, 40(12), 1792-1798
[116] Sattler, CA; Mason, EO, Jr.; Kaplan, SL. Prospective comparison of risk factors and demographic and clinical characteristics of community acquired, methicillin-resistant

versus methicillin-susceptible Staphylococcus aureus infection in children. *Pediatr Infect Dis*, J 2002, 21(10), 910-917

[117] Kaplan, SL; Hulten, KG; Gonzalez, BE; et al. Three-year surveillance of community-acquired Staphylococcus aureus infections in children. *Clin Infect Dis*, 2005, 40(12), 1785-1791

[118] Cherry, DK; Woodwell, D.A. National Ambulatory Medical Care Survey: 2000 summary. *Adv Data*, 2002(328), 1-32

[119] Chant, K; Lowe, D; Rubin, G; et al. Patient-to-patient transmission of HIV in private surgical consulting rooms. *Lancet* 1993, 342(8886 8887), 1548-1549

[120] CDC. Transmission of hepatitis B and C viruses in outpatient settings--New York, Oklahoma, and Nebraska, 2000-2002. *MMWR Morb Mortal Wkly Rep*, 2003;52(38), 901-906

[121] Williams, IT; Perz, JF; Bell, BP. Viral hepatitis transmission in ambulatory health care settings. *Clin Infect Dis*, 2004, 38(11), 1592-1598

[122] Calder, RA; Duclos, P; Wilder, MH; et al. Mycobacterium tuberculosis transmission in a health clinic. *Bull Int Union Tuberc Lung Dis*, 1991, 66(2-3), 103-106

[123] Istre, GR; McKee, PA; West, GR; et al. Measles spread in medical settings: an important focus of disease transmission? *Pediatrics*, 1987, 79(3), 356-358

[124] Jernigan, JA; Lowry, BS; Hayden, FG; et al. Adenovirus type 8 epidemic keratoconjunctivitis in an eye clinic: risk factors and control. *J Infect Dis*, 1993, 167(6), 1307-1313

[125] Fliegel, PE; Weinstein, WM. Rubella outbreak in a prenatal clinic: management and prevention. *Am J Infect Control*, 1982, 10(1), 29-33

[126] Gerberding, J.L. Hospital-onset infections: a patient safety issue. Ann Intern Med 2002, 137(8), 665-670

[127] Leape, LL; Berwick, DM; Bates, DW. What practices will most improve safety? Evidence-based medicine meets patient safety. *JAMA*, 2002, 288(4), 501-507

[128] Burke, J.P. Patient safety: infection control - a problem for patient safety. *N Engl J Med*, 2003;348(7), 651-656

[129] Goldmann, DA; Weinstein, RA; Wenzel, RP; et al. Strategies to Prevent and Control the Emergence and Spread of Antimicrobial-Resistant Microorganisms in Hospitals. A challenge to hospital leadership. *JAMA*, 1996, 275(3), 234-240

[130] Scheckler, WE; Brimhall, D; Buck, AS; et al. Requirements for and essential activities of infection control and epidemiology in hospitals: a consensus panel report. Society for Healthcare Epidemiology of America. *Infect Control Hosp Epidemiol*, 1998, 19(2), 114-124

[131] Stelfox, HT; Bates, DW; Redelmeier, DA. Safety of patients isolated for infection control. *JAMA*, 2003;290(14), 1899-1905

[132] Haley, RW; Culver, DH; White, JW; et al. The efficacy of infection surveillance and control programs in preventing nosocomial infections in US hospitals. *Am J Epidemiol*, 1985, 121(2), 182-205

[133] Turner, JG; Kolenc, KM; Docken, L. Job analysis 1996: Infection control professional. Certification Board in Infection Control and Epidemiology, Inc, 1996 Job Analysis Committee. *Am J Infect Control*, 1999, 27(2), 145-157

[134] Health Canada. Nosocomial and Occupational Infections Section. Development of a resource model for infection prevention and control programs in acute, long term, and

home care settings: conference proceedings of the Infection Prevention and Control Alliance. *AJIC*, 2004, 32, 2-6
[135] Stevenson, KB; Murphy, CL; Samore, MH; et al. Assessing the status of infection control programs in small rural hospitals in the western United States. *Am J Infect Control*, 2004, 32(5), 255-261
[136] Needleman, J; Buerhaus, P; Mattke, S; et al. Nurse-staffing levels and the quality of care in hospitals. *N Engl J Med*, 2002, 346(22), 1715-1722
[137] O'Boyle, C; Jackson, M; Henly, SJ. Staffing requirements for infection control programs in US health care facilities: Delphi project. *Am J Infect Control*, 2002;30(6), 321-333
[138] Robert, J; Fridkin, SK; Blumberg, HM; et al. The influence of the composition of the nursing staff on primary bloodstream infection rates in a surgical intensive care unit. *Infect Control Hosp Epidemiol*, 2000, 21(1), 12-17
[139] Alonso-Echanove, J; Edwards, JR; Richards, MJ; et al. Effect of nurse staffing and antimicrobial-impregnated central venous catheters on the risk for bloodstream infections in intensive care units. *Infect Control Hosp Epidemiol*, 2003, 24(12), 916-925
[140] Teare, EL; Peacock, A. The development of an infection control link-nurse programme in a district general hospital. *J Hosp Infect*, 1996, 34(4), 267-278
[141] Ching, TY; Seto, WH. Evaluating the efficacy of the infection control liaison nurse in the hospital. *J Adv Nurs*, 1990, 15(10), 1128-1131
[142] Pfaller, MA; Herwaldt, LA. The clinical microbiology laboratory and infection control: emerging pathogens, antimicrobial resistance, and new technology. *Clin Infect Dis*, 1997, 25(4), 858-870
[143] Weinstein, RA; Mallison, GF. The role of the microbiology laboratory in surveillance and control of nosocomial infections. *Am J Clin Pathol*, 1978, 69(2), 130-136
[144] Kolmos, HJ; Interaction between the microbiology laboratory and clinician: what the microbiologist can provide. *J Hosp Infect*, 1999, 43 Suppl:S285-291
[145] Sherertz, RJ; Ely, EW; Westbrook, DM; et al. Education of physicians-intraining can decrease the risk for vascular catheter infection. *Ann Intern Med*, 2000, 132(8), 641-648
[146] Lynch, P; Cummings, MJ; Roberts, PL; et al. Implementing and evaluating a system of generic infection precautions: body substance isolation. *Am J Infect Control*, 1990, 18(1), 1-12
[147] Courington, KR; Patterson, SL; Howard, RJ. Universal precautions are not universally followed. *Arch Surg*, 1991, 126(1), 93-96
[148] Henry, K; Campbell, S; Collier, P; et al. Compliance with universal precautions and needle handling and disposal practices among emergency department staff at two community hospitals. *Am J Infect Control*, 1994, 22(3), 129-137
[149] Eustis, TC; Wright, SW; Wrenn, KD; et al. Compliance with recommendations for universal precautions among prehospital providers. *Ann Emerg Med*, 1995, 25(4), 512-515
[150] Helfgott, AW; Taylor-Burton, J; Garcini, FJ; et al. Compliance with universal precautions: knowledge and behavior of residents and students in a department of obstetrics and gynecology. *Infect Dis Obstet Gynecol*, 1998, 6(3), 123-128
[151] Moore, S; Goodwin, H; Grossberg, R; et al. Compliance with universal precautions among pediatric residents. *Arch Pediatr Adolesc Med*, 1998, 152(6), 554-557

[152] Williams, CO; Campbell, S; Henry, K; et al. Variables influencing worker compliance with universal precautions in the emergency department. *Am J Infect Control*, 1994, 22(3), 138-148

[153] Brooks, AJ; Phipson, M; Potgieter, A; et al. Education of the trauma team: video evaluation of the compliance with universal barrier precautions in resuscitation. *Eur J Surg*, 1999, 165(12), 1125-1128

[154] Harbarth, S; Siegrist, CA; Schira, JC; et al. Influenza immunization: improving compliance of healthcare workers. *Infect Control Hosp Epidemiol*, 1998, 19(5), 337-342

[155] Martinello, RA; Jones, L; Topal, JE. Correlation between healthcare workers' knowledge of influenza vaccine and vaccine receipt. *Infect Control Hosp Epidemiol*, 2003, 24(11):845-7

[156] Jarvis WR. Handwashing-the Semmelweis lesson forgotten? Lancet 1994;344(8933), 1311-1312

[157] Daniels, IR; Rees, BI. Handwashing: simple, but effective. *Ann R Coll Surg Engl*, 1999, 81, 117-118

[158] Labarraque, AG. *Instructions and observations regarding the use of the chlorides of soda and lime*, Porter J, (ed.). [French] New Haven, CT: Baldwin and Treadway, 1829

[159] Maharaj, D. Puerperal Pyrexia: A Review. Part I. *Obstet Gynecol Surv* 2007, 62(6), 393-399

[160] Raju, TN. Ignac Semmelweiss and the etiology of fetal and neonatal sepsis. *J Perinatol* 1999, 19, 307–310

[161] Dunn, PM. Ignac Semmelweiss (1818–1865) of Budapest and the prevention of puerperal fever. *Arch Dis Child Fetal Neonatal Ed*, 2005, 90, F345–F348

[162] Daniels, IR. Historical perspectives on health. Semmelweiss: a lesson to relearn? *J R Soc Health*, 1998, 118, 367–370.

[163] Centers for Disease Control and Prevention. Guideline for Hand Hygiene in Health-Care Settings: Recommendations of the Healthcare Infection Control Practices Advisory Committee and the HICPAC/SHEA/APIC/IDSA Hand Hygiene Task Force. *MMWR*, 2002, 51(No. RR- 16)

[164] Larson, EL; Cronquist, AB; Whittier, S; et al. Differences in skin flora between inpatients and chronically ill patients. *Heart Lung*, 2000, 29, 298–305

[165] Lowbury, EJL. Gram-negative bacilli on the skin. *Br J Dermatol*, 1969;81(suppl 1):55–61

[166] Sanderson, PJ; Weissler, S. Recovery of coliforms from the hands of nurses and patients: activities leading to contamination. *J Hosp Infect*, 1992, 21, 85–93

[167] Noble, WC. Dispersal of skin microorganisms. *Br J Dermatol* 1975, 93, 477–485

[168] Walter, CW; Kundsin, RB; Shilkret, MA; et al. Spread of staphylococci to the environment. *Antibiotics Annual*, 1959, 952–957

[169] Samore, MH; Venkataraman, L; DeGirolami, PC; et al. Clinical and molecular epidemiology of sporadic and clustered cases of nosocomial *Clostridium difficile* diarrhea. *Am J Med*, 1996, 100, 32–40

[170] Patrick, DR; Findon, G; Miller, TE. Residual moisture determines the level of touch-contact-associated bacterial transfer following hand washing. *Epidemiol Infect*, 1997, 119, 319–325

[171] Pittet, D; Hugonnet, S; Harbarth, S; et al. Effectiveness of a hospital-wide programme to improve compliance with hand hygiene. *Lancet*, 2000, 356, 1307–1312

[172] Edel, E; Houston, S; Kennedy, V; et al. Impact of a 5-minute scrub on the microbial flora found on artificial, polished, or natural fingernails of operating room personnel. *Nurs Res*, 1998, 47(1), 54-59

[173] Hedderwick, SA ; McNeil, SA ; Lyons, MJ ; et al. Pathogenic organisms associated with artificial fingernails worn by healthcare workers. *Infect Control Hosp Epidemiol*, 2000, 21(8), 505-509

[174] CDC. Guideline for Hand Hygiene in Health-Care Settings: Recommendations of the Healthcare Infection Control Practices Advisory Committee and the HICPAC/SHEA/APIC/IDSA Hand Hygiene Task Force. *MMWR*, 2002, 51(16)(RR-16), 1-44

[175] Parry, MF; Grant, B; Yukna, M, et al. Candida osteomyelitis and diskitis after spinal surgery: an outbreak that implicates artificial nail use. *Clin Infect Dis*, 2001, 32(3), 352-357

[176] Boszczowski, I; Nicoletti, C; Puccini, DM; et al. Outbreak of extended spectrum beta-lactamase-producing Klebsiella pneumoniae infection in a neonatal intensive care unit related to onychomycosis in a health care worker. *Pediatr Infect Dis J*, 2005, 24(7), 648-650

[177] Trick, WE; Vernon, MO; Hayes, RA; et al. Impact of ring wearing on hand contamination and comparison of hand hygiene agents in a hospital. *Clin Infect Dis*, 2003, 36(11), 1383-1390

[178] Korniewicz, DM; McLeskey, SW. Latex allergy and gloving standards. *Semin Perioper Nurs*, 1998, 7(4), 216-221

[179] Ranta, PM; Ownby, DR. A review of natural-rubber latex allergy in healthcare workers. *Clin Infect Dis*, 2004, 38(2), 252-256

[180] Korniewicz, DM; Kirwin, M; Cresci, K; et al. Barrier protection with examination gloves: double versus single. *Am J Infect Control*, 1994, 22(1), 12-15

[181] CDC. Recommendations for preventing the spread of vancomycin resistance. Recommendations of the Hospital Infection Control Practices Advisory Committee (HICPAC). *MMWR Recomm Rep*, 1995, 44 (RR12): 1-13

[182] Olsen, RJ; Lynch, P; Coyle, MB; et al. Examination gloves as barriers to hand contamination in clinical practice. *JAMA*, 1993, 270(3), 350-353

[183] Doebbeling, BN, Pfaller, MA; Houston, AK; et al. Removal of nosocomial pathogens from the contaminated glove. Implications for glove reuse and handwashing. *Ann Intern Med*, 1988, 109(5), 394-398

[184] Serrano, CW; Wright, JW; Newton, ER. Surgical glove perforation in obstetrics. *Obstet Gynecol*, 1991, 77, 525-527

[185] Boyce, JM ; Mermel, LA; Zervos, MJ ; et al. Controlling vancomycin resistant enterococci. *Infect Control Hosp Epidemiol*, 1995, 16(11), 634-637

[186] National Institute for Occupational Safety and Health. Eye protection for infection control. 2004. Available at: www.cdc.gov/niosh/topics/eye/eye-infectious.html Accessed on August 12 2008

[187] Loeb, M; McGeer, A; Henry, B; et al. SARS among critical care nurses, Toronto. *Emerg Infect Dis*, 2004, 10(2), 251-255

[188] Garibaldi, RA; Maglio, S; Lerer, T; et al. Comparison of nonwoven and woven gown and drape fabric to prevent intraoperative wound contamination and postoperative infection. *Am J Surg*, 1986, 152(5), 505-509
[189] Muller, W; Jiru, P; Mach, R; et al. The use of disposable draping materials in the operating room and its effect on the postoperative wound infection rate. *Wein Klin Wochenschr*, 1989, 101, 837-842
[190] Dineen, P; Drusin, L. Epidemics of postoperative wound infections associated with hair carriers. *Lancet*, 1973;2(7839), 1157-1159
[191] Ha'eri, GB. Wiley, AM. The efficacy of standard surgical face masks: an investigation using "tracer particles." *Clin Orthop*, 1980, 148, 160-162
[192] Moylan, JA; Balish, E; Chan, J. Intraoperative bacterial transmission. *Surg Forum*, 1974, 25, 29-30
[193] Mastro, TD; Farley, TA; Elliott, JA; et al. An outbreak of surgical-wound infections due to group A streptococcus carried on the scalp. *N Engl J Med*, 1990, 323, 968-972
[194] Humphreys, H; Marshall, RJ; Ricketts, VE; et al. Theatre over-shoes do not reduce operating theatre floor bacterial counts. *J Hosp Infect*, 1991, 17, 117-123
[195] Weightman, NC; Banfield, KR. Protective over-shoes are unnecessary in a day surgery unit. *J Hosp Infect*, 1994, 28, 1-3
[196] Do, AN; Ciesielski, CA; Metler, RP; et al. Occupationally acquired human immunodeficiency virus (HIV) infection: national case surveillance data during 20 years of the HIV epidemic in the United States. *Infect Control Hosp Epidemiol*, 2003, 24(2), 86-96
[197] CDC. Workbook for Designing, Implementing, and Evaluating a Sharps Injury Prevention Program. Available at: http://www.cdc.gov/sharpssafety/pdf/Workbook-Complete.pdf Accessed on August 20 2008
[198] Mulin, B; Rouget, C; Clement, C; et al. Association of private isolation rooms with ventilator-associated Acinetobacter baumanii pneumonia in a surgical intensive-care unit. *Infect Control Hosp Epidemiol*, 1997, 18(7), 499-503
[199] Isaacs, D; Dickson, H; O'Callaghan, C; et al. Handwashing and cohorting in prevention of hospital acquired infections with respiratory syncytial virus. *Arch Dis Child*, 1991, 66(2):227-231
[200] Mayer, RA; Geha, RC; Helfand, MS; et al. Role of fecal incontinence in contamination of the environment with vancomycin-resistant enterococci. *Am J Infect Control*, 2003, 31(4), 221-225
[201] Bruce, BB; Blass, MA; Blumberg, HM; et al. Risk of Cryptosporidium parvum transmission between hospital roommates. *Clin Infect Dis*, 2000, 31(4), 947-950
[202] Ford-Jones, EL; Mindorff, CM; Gold, R; et al. The incidence of viralassociated diarrhea after admission to a pediatric hospital. *Am J Epidemiol*, 1990, 131(4), 711-718
[203] Austin, DJ; Bonten, MJ; Weinstein, RA; et al. Vancomycin-resistant enterococci in intensive-care hospital settings: transmission dynamics, persistence, and the impact of infection control programs. *Proc Natl Acad Sci USA*, 1999, 96(12), 6908-6913
[204] CDC. Update: Severe Acute Respiratory Syndrome. *MMWR*, 2003, 52(23), 547-550
[205] Hota, B. Contamination, disinfection, and cross-colonization: are hospital surfaces reservoirs for nosocomial infection? *Clin Infect Dis*, 2004, 39(8), 1182-1189
[206] Rutala, WA; Weber, DJ. Disinfection and sterilization in health care facilities: what clinicians need to know. *Clin Infect Dis*, 2004, 39(5), 702-709

[207] Wilcox, MH; Fawley, WN; Wigglesworth, N; et al. Comparison of the effect of detergent versus hypochlorite cleaning on environmental contamination and incidence of Clostridium difficile infection. *J Hosp Infect*, 2003, 54(2), 109-114

[208] Bernards, AT; Harinck, HI; Dijkshoorn, L; et al. Persistent Acinetobacter baumannii? Look inside your medical equipment. *Infect Control Hosp Epidemiol*, 2004, 25(11), 1002-1004

[209] Bures, S; Fishbain, JT; Uyehara, CF; et al. Computer keyboards and faucet handles as reservoirs of nosocomial pathogens in the intensive care unit. *Am J Infect Control*, 2000, 28(6), 465-471

[210] Mahoney, FJ; Stewart, K; Hu, H; et al. Progress toward the elimination of hepatitis B virus transmission among health care workers in the United States. *Arch Intern Med*, 1997, 157(22), 2601-2605

[211] Gladstone, JL; Millian, SJ. Rubella exposure in an obstetric clinic. *Obstet Gynecol*, 1981, 57(2), 182-186

[212] Wilde, JA; McMillan, JA; Serwint, J; et al. Effectiveness of influenza vaccine in health care professionals: a randomized trial. *JAMA*, 1999, 281(10), 908-913.

In: Cross Infections: Types, Causes and Prevention
Editors: Jin Dong and Xun Liang
ISBN: 978-1-60741-467-4
© 2009 Nova Science Publishers, Inc.

Chapter II

The Role of Panton Valentine Leukocidin as a Virulence Factor in Community-Associated Methicillin-Resistant *Staphylococcus aureus*

Kunyan Zhang
Centre for Antimicrobial Resistance, University of Calgary/Alberta Health Services/Calgary Laboratory Services, Calgary, Alberta, Canada

Abstract

Newly-emerging community-associated methicillin resistant *Staphylococcus aureus* (CA-MRSA) strains have caused serious community-acquired infections in otherwise healthy children, athletes, and young adults lacking typical risk factors for nosocomial MRSA acquisition. The most commonly encountered clinical manifestations include severe skin and soft tissue infections and necrotizing pneumonia. These strains often carry the Panton-Valentine leukocidin (PVL) genes. PVL is a bi-component, pore-forming leukotoxin, recently classified as a member of the family of synergohymenotropic toxins, which causes leukocyte destruction and tissue necrosis but also possesses chemotactic and proinflammatory properties. However, the specific role of PVL as a major virulence factor in CA-MRSA infections has been controversial. Recent studies of PVL knockout strains of CA-MRSA USA300 and USA400 in murine sepsis and abscess models have shown that PVL(-) strains were as lethal and virulent as wild-type strains and caused comparable skin diseases, and that lysis of human neutrophils and pathogen survival after phagocytosis were similar between wild-type and mutant strains. However, a study using a laboratory stain overexpressing plasmid-encoded PVL gene in a mouse acute pneumonia model indicated that PVL alone is sufficient to cause necrotizing pneumonia. But another study using a different murine model of staphylococcal pneumonia that mimics clinicopathologic features of human disease did not support PVL having any impact in this model, and anti-PVL serum failed to protect mice from staphylococcal pneumonia. In addition, recent studies of human CA-MRSA infections in community and hospital patients in our health care region over a six-year period identified the co-existence of two USA400 (a major clonal group of CA-MRSA) sibling strains with and without PVL genes. These strains shared identical genotypic, phenotypic and clinical characteristics. PCR and sequence analysis indicated that the PVL carrying prophage ϕSa2mw was present in PVL(+) but absent in PVL(-) USA400 isolates. These findings provided the first direct human evidence that PVL genes are not necessarily the key determinants associated with the increased dissemination of CA-MRSA strains. We conducted further experimental studies using various in vitro cell culture and animal models of these sibling strains and found that PVL(+) and PVL(-) USA400 strains exhibited identical virulence characteristics in these models. Combined with data from murine models, the weight of the evidence currently suggests that the genomic milieu rather than the PVL gene plays the most significant role in the virulence and widespread dissemination of CA-MRSA.

Introduction

Staphylococcus aureus is a leading cause of disease ranging from mild skin and soft tissue infections and food poisoning to life-threatening illnesses such as deep post-surgical infections, septicaemia, endocarditis, hemorrhagic pneumonia, and toxic shock syndrome [1-4]. This organism has a remarkable ability to accumulate additional antibiotic resistance determinants, resulting in the formation of multiply-drug-resistant strains. Methicillin, the first semi-synthetic penicillin to be developed, was introduced in 1959 to overcome the problem of penicillin-resistant *S. aureus* due to β-lactamase (penicillinase) production [2]. However, methicillin-resistant *S. aureus* (MRSA) strains were identified soon after the introduction of methicillin [5,6]. MRSA has acquired and integrated into its genome a 21-67kb mobile genetic element, termed the staphylococcal cassette chromosome *mec* (SCC*mec*) that harbours the methicillin resistance (*mecA*) gene and other antibiotic resistance determinants [7-12]. The *mecA* gene encodes an altered additional low affinity penicillin-binding protein (PBP2a) [13-15] that confers broad resistance to almost all penicillin-related compounds including cephalosporins and carbapenems, which are currently the most potent broad-spectrum drugs available. Since then, strains of MRSA have spread and become established as major nosocomial pathogens (hospital-associated, HA-MRSA) worldwide [16-19]. The dominant worldwide HA-MRSA clones/lineages include the Iberian (ST247-MRSA-IA), Brazilian/Hungarian (ST239-MRSA-III), New York/Japan (ST5-MRSA-II), Pediatric (ST5-MRSA-IV), EMRSA-16 (ST36-MRSA-II), EMRSA-15 (ST22-MRSA-IV), and Berlin (ST45-MRSA-IV) clones [20-23]. They have been responsible for major outbreaks of infection in hospitalized individuals, nursing home patients, chronically ill individuals, and prison inmates.

While MRSA continues to be a major cause of hospital-associated infections, recently, MRSA has rapidly emerged as an important cause of community-associated infection, referred to as community-associated MRSA (CA-MRSA) [24-27]. These newly-emerging CA-MRSA strains are causing serious community-acquired infections/outbreaks in otherwise healthy children, athletes, and other individuals lacking typical risk factors for nosocomial MRSA acquisition [28-46]. CA-MRSA infection is now a leading cause of disease in otherwise healthy individuals [47, 48]. For instance, the majority of all skin and soft tissue infections in patients presenting to emergency departments in the United States were caused by CA-MRSA [49]. The most dominant and aggressive CA-MRSA strain, USA300, has reportedly spread into and within the hospital environment with subsequent acquisition of multiple drug resistance genes, and is now emerging as a worldwide pandemic MRSA strain [50-60]. In October 2007, the CDC reported in its first overall estimate of invasive disease caused by MRSA that more than 90,000 Americans may develop potentially deadly infections each year by this organism, primarily (67%) USA300 isolates, indicating that "the number of deaths caused by MRSA exceeds the number of deaths attributable to HIV/AIDS in US" [44]. Hence, the emerging spread of these CA-MRSA strains poses a great threat to public health.

Current evidence from molecular studies points to an intra- and inter-continental spread of a limited number of CA-MRSA clones carrying Panton-Valentine leukocidin (PVL) genes that are genetically distinct from epidemic nosocomial strains [27, 61]. These include ST1-MRSA-IV, ST8-MRSA-IV and ST59-MRSA-IV strains in the USA; ST80-MRSA-IV strain in France, Switzerland and other European countries; ST30-MRSA-IV strain in Oceania; and ST93-MRSA-IV strain in Australia [27, 62]. Although diversity and variation in their genomic and antibiogram backgrounds exist, virtually all of these newly-emerging CA-MRSA strains carry the PVL virulence determinant and a novel small mobile SCC*mec* type IV or V genetic element [27, 45, 49, 63-65] that, when compared with larger *SCCmec* types (I, II and III) prevalent in HA-MRSA, exhibit a high degree of horizontal transmissibility [14, 66].

There is a strong epidemiological association between CA-MRSA infections and the presence of PVL, suggesting that PVL may be, at least, a marker for CA-MRSA [27, 67]. PVL's biological role, however, is not yet established. There is currently no direct evidence to suggest that PVL plays a significant role in the epidemiology and pathogenesis of CA-MRSA infections. Meanwhile, several recent reports have provided conflicting views of the role of PVL in CA-MRSA infections [68-81]. This chapter summarizes the history and our current evidence and understanding of the epidemiology and molecular biology of PVL in CA-MRSA infections.

PVL

PVL, an *S. aureus*-specific exotoxin initially designated "substance leukocidine" due to its ability to lyse leukocytes, was first discovered by van deVelde in 1894 [82]. Panton and Valentine [83] later associated the leukotoxin with skin and soft tissue infection in 1932, long before MRSA was of clinical concern. The PVL toxin was purified in 1991 from an *S. aureus* strain V8 (ATCC49775) isolated from a patient with chronic furunculosis [84]. The toxin consists of two polypeptides, S- (slow-eluted) and F- (fast-eluted) components, based on their elution profiles through cation-exchange chromatography [85-87]. The genes for the toxin were later cloned and sequenced in 1995 by Prevost et al., and were renamed PVL (*LukS*-PV and *LukF*-PV) to distinguish them from other homologous leukotoxins with hemolytic activities [88]. It has been well established that PVL genes (*luk*S- and *luk*F-PV) are encoded by a phage that integrates into the *S. aureus* chromosome. To date, there are five phages that have been reported to carry PVL genes, including ϕPVL [89], ϕSLT [90], ϕSa2mw [91], ϕ108PVL [92] and, most recently, ϕSa2958 [93]. The presence or absence of the PVL genes in clinical isolates can be detected by PCR [94-99].

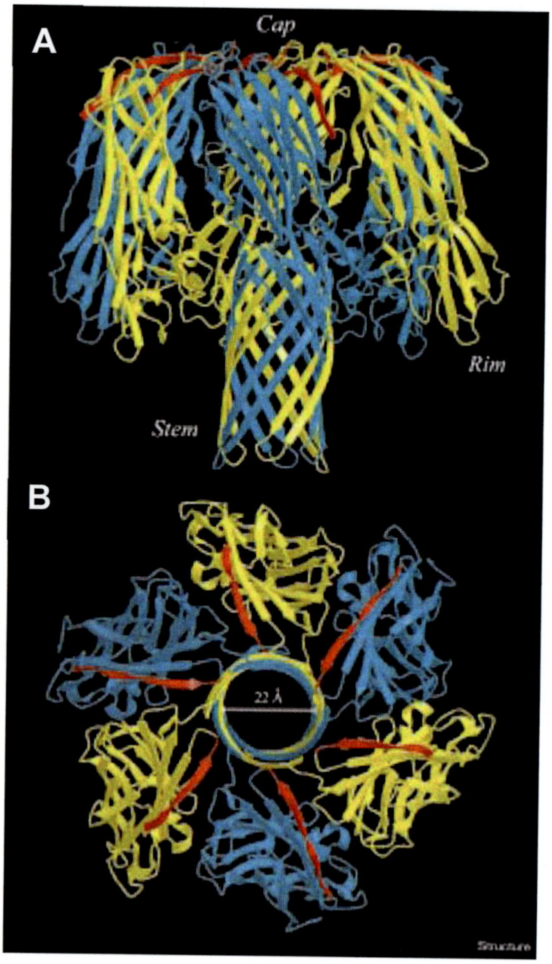

Figure 1. Molecular model of heterohexameric PVL. (A) View perpendicular to the sixfold axis. The LukF and LukS subunits are shown in blue and yellow, respectively; the N termini are shown in red. (B) View down the sixfold axis from the top of the cap. (Adapted from Pedelacq et al. 1999 [101].)

PVL is now recognized as a bi-component, pore-forming leukotoxin and was recently classified as a member of the family of synergohymenotropic toxins that induces pores in the membranes of cells (Figure 1) [100, 101]. Two proteins (polypeptides), LukS-PV and LukF-PV of PVL (33 and 34 kDa in size, respectively), act together as subunits, assembling in the membrane of host defense cells, particularly polymorph nuclear cells, monocytes and macrophages [88, 102]. The subunits fit together and form a ring with a central pore through which cell contents leak and which acts as a superantigen [87, 88, 102, 103]. It causes leukocyte destruction and tissue necrosis, and possesses chemotactic and proinflammatory properties [100, 104]. Purified PVL was reported to induce severe inflammatory lesion when injected intradermally in rabbits, leading to capillary dilation, infiltration of polymorphonuclear cells, and skin necrosis [105], contributing to the hypothesis that this toxin has a role in skin and soft-tissue infections. However, early reports have concluded that PVL alone is not a toxic substance because intravenous injection of PVL in rabbits resulted in granulocytopenia followed by a marked granulocytosis but was not lethal [106].

PVL Associated with Skin and Soft Tissue Infection and in CA-MRSA Infection

PVL can be harbored in both MSSA and MRSA, but was found in <5% of *S. aureus* clinical isolates around the world before the emergence of CA-MRSA [27, 104, 107]. Provost et al. [104] reported that PVL was detected in fewer than 5% of the isolates in a general hospital. In accordance with the aforementioned activities of purified PVL, PVL-positivity of *S. aureus* strains was found to be associated with primary skin infections such as furunculosis, and severe necrotizing pneumonia [104]. The clinical importance of PVL was further demonstrated in a study of *S. aureus* infections which occurred between 1986 and 1998 in France [96]. A collection of 172 *S. aureus* strains was screened for PVL genes by PCR. PVL genes were detected in 93% of strains associated with furunculosis and in 85% of those associated with severe necrotic hemorrhagic pneumonia (all community-acquired) [96]. This study revealed eight cases of community-acquired pneumonia caused by PVL-positive *S. aureus* strains, six of which with a fatal outcome [96]. The patients involved were all immunocompetent children and young adults, and each of them presented with a preceding influenza-like syndrome before developing pneumonia [96].

Furthermore, Vandenesch et al. [27] performed a study in which the presence of 24 virulence factors and the SCC*mec* types in 117 CA-MRSA isolates from a large number of countries worldwide was investigated. This study showed that although diversity and variation in their genomic and antibiogram backgrounds existed, virtually all of these newly emerging CA-MRSA strains carried the PVL virulence determinant and a novel small mobile SCC*mec* type IV genetic element [27].

Although the molecular basis for the enhanced virulence compared to HA-MRSA is not known, there is a strong association between CA-MRSA infections and the presence of PVL, suggesting that PVL may be a marker for CA-MRSA [27, 67]. The presence of PVL in *S. aureus* has been reported to be associated with increased disease severity, ranging from cutaneous infections requiring surgical drainage to severe chronic osteomyelitis, deadly necrotizing pneumonia and a recently described syndrome of severe septicaemia with Waterhouse-Friderichsen syndrome [45, 49, 64, 65, 107-116]. These observations, however, do not exclude the possibility of coincidental co-presence of PVL genes in a virulent genomic background of CA-MRSA strains. There is currently little direct evidence to suggest that PVL plays a significant role in the epidemiology and pathogenesis of CA-MRSA infections.

Conflicting Views of the Role of PVL in *In Vitro* and *In Vivo* Animal Experiments

Several studies have demonstrated that PVL could cause dermonecrosis in animal models [88, 117]. However, several recent reports have provided conflicting views of the role of PVL in the pathogenesis of CA-MRSA disease.

Voyich et al. [68] studied the PVL knockout isogenic strains of USA300 (LAC) and USA400 (MW2) in mouse sepsis (CD1 Swiss) and abscess (hairless Crl:SKH1-hrBR) models and showed that PVL(-) strains were as lethal and virulent as wild-type strains and caused comparable skin diseases, and that lysis of human neutrophils and pathogen survival after phagocytosis were similar between wild-type and mutant strains. They concluded that PVL is not the major virulence determinant of CA-MRSA [68].

However, in an investigation using laboratory MRSA strain RN6390 and RN6390 variants expressing either native phage- or plasmid-encoded PVL in a BALB/c model of *S. aureus* pneumonia, Labandeira-Rey et al. [69] reported that PVL promoted staphylococcal lung infection and PVL alone was sufficient to cause necrotizing pneumonia in this mouse acute pneumonia model. Importantly, in this system, death was evident only when PVL was expressed from a plasmid, presumably yielding high levels of PVL expression [69].

In contrast to the above Labandeira-Rey et al. observations, another study using a different murine model of staphylococcal pneumonia that mimics the clinicopathologic features of human disease did not support PVL having any impact in this model and anti-PVL serum failed to protect mice from staphylococcal pneumonia [70]. Bubeck Wardenburg et al. evaluated LAC and MW2 clinical isolates and PVL-knockout mutants in a C57BL/6J model of *S. aureus* pneumonia and demonstrated that wild-type and mutant strains were equally virulent when death, the bacterial load in infected tissue, or pathologic evidence of disease was evaluated as the experimental end point [70]. Part of the reasons for these conflicting reports may be due to the different host genetic backgrounds of mouse use, which may alter susceptibility/response to the PVL toxin, as dictated by the genetic makeup of the mouse strain. To exclude this possibility, the same group [71] expanded their studies by assessing the contribution of PVL in the genetic background of BALB/c mice, which is the same genetic background mouse as Labandeira-Rey et al. [69] used. But this study reported that PVL does not contribute to the pathogenesis of staphylococcal infection of BALB/c mice either [71].

Most recently, Diep et al. [72] conducted microarray and proteomic analyses on (using) the wild-type parental and isogenic PVL-deletion strains of USA300 (LAC and SF8300) and USA400 (MW2) and revealed that PVL does not alter gene or protein expression, therefore demonstrating that any contribution of PVL to CA-MRSA pathogenesis is not mediated through interference of global gene regulatory networks. To test whether PVL contributes to pathogenesis of bacteremia directly, Diep et al. [72] developed a rabbit bacteremia model of CA-MRSA infection to evaluate the effects of PVL, an animal species whose granulocytes are more sensitive to the effects of PVL compared with the mouse. They used this rabbit model to compare wild-type parental and isogenic PVL mutant strain pairs using a competition design. Rabbits were coinfected with a mixture of parent and PVL-mutant strains in an approximate 1:1 ratio. Normalized ratios of the parent to PVL mutant, representing competition indexes, were determined in organs harvested from rabbits that succumbed to infection or moribund rabbits with end stage bacteremia. The competition indexes in the rabbit lung, spleen, kidney and blood did not differ significantly from the null effect value of 0 between the wild-type and the isogenic strain pairs, indicating no contribution of PVL to bacterial colonization and persistence at the end stages of bacteremia in the competition model [72]. However, when used a single-strain infection rabbit bacteremia model, they found that at 24 and 48 hours post infection, PVL appears to play a modest, but measurable role in pathogenesis during the early stages of bacteremic seeding of the kidney (only in kidney but not in other organs), the target organ from which bacteria were not cleared. However, the early survival advantage of this USA300 strain conferred by PVL was lost by 72 hours post infection [72]. These data seem to be consistent with the clinical presentation of rapid-onset, fulminant infection that has been associated with PVL-positive CA-MRSA strains. Therefore they suggested that PVL may have a modest and transient positive effect in the acute phase of bacteremia, providing evidence that PVL contributes to CA-MRSA pathogenesis [72].

However, the arguing point is how relevant were the animal models used to measure the impact of PVL in human staphylococcal infections [73, 74]. For example, mouse leukocytes are not lysed by PVL as they are in rabbits and humans [75]. Also, in the mouse sepsis model, mice are relatively resistant to intravenous bacterial challenges, which necessitates the use of high concentrations over relatively short periods of time [76]. The immediate response to bacterial cell-wall constituents in the mouse model is likely to obscure the contributions of secreted toxins [74]. Thus, direct data from the human population may present more relevant evidence.

Genetic Diversity among PVL (+) *S. Aureus* Isolates

The Calgary Health Region (CHR) is one of Canada's largest integrated urban healthcare regions and provides medical services for a population of about 1.25 million people with 1900 acute care beds housed in 4 acute care facilities and several community health centers in the Calgary area including the cities of Calgary and Airdrie and about 20 nearby smaller outlying communities. Calgary Laboratory Services (CLS) provides centralized diagnostic microbiology services for the entire CHR.

In order to determine the PVL prevalence in natural populations of staphylococci and their genetic profiles, we conducted a retrospective study based on testing of our local clinical isolates collected in the CHR over the last 16 years from 1989 to 2004. Randomly selected clinical isolates from frozen collections of MSSA, MRSA and coagulase-negative staphylococci (CoNS) were tested for PVL genes using our multiplex PCR assay which detects the staphylococcal virulence marker PVL genes with simultaneous discrimination of methicillin-susceptible from methicillin-resistant staphylococci [97]. PVL+ isolates were fingerprinted by pulsed field gel electrophoresis (PFGE) [118] and further characterized with SCC*mec* typing using a multiplex PCR assay to classify the isolates as type and subtypes I, II, III, IVa, IVb, IVc, IVd, and V [66], multilocus sequence typing (MLST) [119], staphylococcal protein A (*spa*) typing [120] and accessory gene regulator (*agr*) typing [121] as previously described. The eBURST algorithm [122, 123] was used to discern the descent patterns of clonal complexes. Antibiotic susceptibility was determined by standard procedures.

Our results revealed that the mean PVL+ rate was 1.6% and 1.4% for MRSA (n=1259) and MSSA (n=1031), respectively, with slight yearly variation (excluding isolates from a clonal outbreak of PVL+ CA-MRSA USA300 strain in 2004 [43]). No CoNS (n=448) were PVL+. The PVL genes existed not only in the currently described CA-MRSA clones including ST1-MRSA-IV (USA400 strain), ST8-MRSA-IV (USA300 strain), ST59-MRSA-IV, ST80-MRSA-IV and ST30-MRSA-IV, but also in MSSA strains (ST5, ST22, ST25, ST30, ST39, ST59, ST121, ST217, ST942). Interestingly, we also found PVL genes in strains with genomic backgrounds similar to those of typical epidemic HA-MRSA, being frequently associated with SCC*mec* type II and III, and MLST types ST5, ST30, ST22, ST45 and ST105. The eBURST analyses did not reveal clear descent evolution of these PVL+ strains. The antibiotic resistant profiles of these PVL+ isolates were closely associated with SCC*mec* types (r=0.988; p<0.01) rather than PVL genes (Figure 2; [77]).

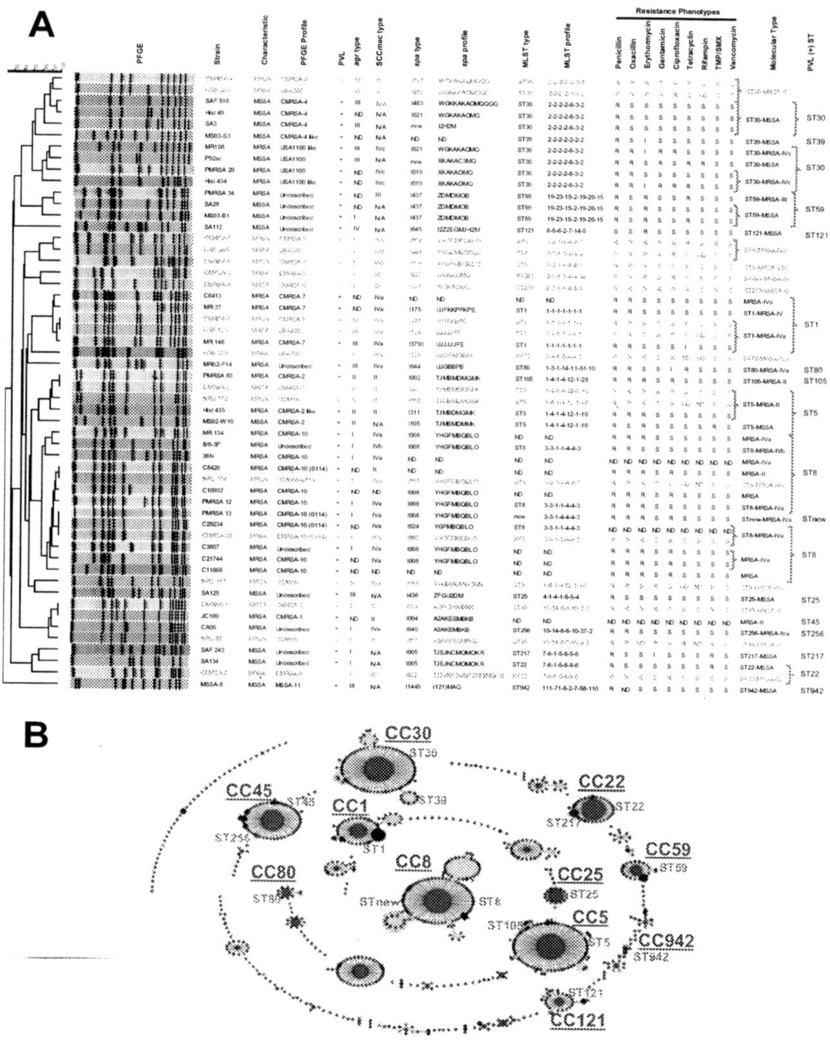

Figure 2. Genetic Diversity Among PVL-positive *Staphylococcus aureus* clinical Isolates over 16 Years (1989-2004) in a Large Canadian Healthcare Region. (A) Molecular, Genomic and antimicrobial susceptibility profiles of representative PVL-positive strains. Highlights of the utility of PFGE (pulsed field gel electrophoresis), PVL (Panton Valentine leukocidin) genes, *agr* (accessory gene regulator) typing, SCC*mec* (staphylococcal cassette chromosome *mec*) typing, *spa* (staphylococcal protein A) typing, MLST (multilocus sequence typing), and antimicrobial resistance phenotypes for strain characterization. (B) The eBURST analyses did not reveal clear descent evolution of these PVL+ strains. The eBURST algorithm compare our MLST data (16 ST types) with the international MLST database (no. isolates=2329; no. STs=919; No. groups=48; updated December 9, 2008). The MLST data was divided into groups of related clonal complexes (CC), the founding genotype of each clonal complex was predicted, and the bootstrap support for the assignment was computed (re-sampling for bootstrapping=1000).

The results of our study provide the first indirect evidence from the population-based study that PVL genes are not necessarily the key determinant(s) associated with newly emerging CA-MRSA clones and suggest that the genomic milieu may play a greater role in the emergence of current CA-MRSA infections/outbreaks [77].

Since then, the epidemiological data from the population-based studies that did not support PVL directly contributes to widespread dissemination of CA-MRSA clones began to appear (emerge), although there are still only a few. For instance, Diep et al. [78] studied 34 virulence-gene content (including PVL) of a representative sample of MRSA isolates collected from inpatients and outpatients over 8.5 years of laboratory-based surveillance in San Francisco and reported that not PVL but the other virulence determinants have made to the evolution of contemporary epidemic CA-MRSA strains, suggesting the PVL genes appear not to be essential for the evolution of community-associated strains of MRSA (78). Rossney et al. [79] investigated MRSA isolates including CA-MRSA, health care-associated MRSA and HA-MRSA from Ireland for the carriage of PVL and determined the genotypic characteristics of all PVL-positive isolates identified. This study, similar to our study, revealed the diverse genotypes of PVL-positive MRSA in Ireland and suggested that PVL is a poor (not a reliable) marker for CA-MRSA [79]. Moreover, Monecke et al. [80] also observed high diversity of PVL-positive MSSA strains in Germany and some of which (agrI/ST152, agrIII/ST80 and agrIII/ST96) are closely resembled known epidemic CA-MRSA strains. These findings indicate that the current rise in PVL-positive CA-MRSA could be caused by the dissemination of novel SCC*mec* elements (Type IV and V) among pre-existing PVL-positive strains, rather than by the spread of PVL phages among MRSA strains [80]. Recently, Tomita et al. [124] reported two cases of severe necrotizing pneumonia caused by PVL-negative CA-MRSA infections in Japan. Unlike the severe CA-MRSA cases in western countries, PVL genes were not detected in these cases, the authors suggested that factors other than PVL had a significant effect on the severity of necrotizing pneumonia.

However, these indirect evidences of the epidemiological data (high genetic diversity of PVL-positive MRSA and MSSA strains from the population-based studies) alone are insufficient to establish whether PVL directly contributes to currently widespread dissemination of CA-MRSA strains. Direct evidence would be more compelling.

Co-Existence of PVL (+) and PVL (-) CA-MRSA USA400 Sibling Strains

The USA400 strain (ST1-MRSA-IV) is a major clonal group of CA-MRSA currently circulating in the USA and Canada and one that has been implicated in outbreaks of community-onset infections associated with serious morbidity and mortality [25, 41, 125].

We conducted a retrospective study on a natural population of MRSA clinical isolates recovered from patients in a large Canadian healthcare region during a six-year period (2000-2005) and identified the co-existence of PVL (+)/(-) sibling USA400 strains with the PVL (-) strain dominant (Figure 3) [81]. Sequencing and molecular studies indicated that the prophage ϕSa2mw which carrys the PVL genes was present in PVL (+) strain but missing in PVL (-) strain (Figure 4). Both PVL (+) and (-) strains shared identical MLST (ST1), SCC*mec* (IVa), *spa* (t128), and *agr* (III) profiles (Figure 5), and possessed the same toxin, adhesion and exoenzyme virulence gene profiles, carrying *sea*, *sec* and *seh* but lacking TSST-1 (Table 1), and had similar resistance phenotypes (Figure 5) and clinical characteristics (Table 2).

This work provides the first direct evidence from a natural population of MRSA clinical isolates that supports the hypothesis that PVL genes are not the key determinants associated with the increasing dissemination of CA-MRSA strains, suggesting that the genomic milieu, particularly the repertoire of virulence and resistance genes, may play a greater role in this regard. This study had been presented at the 106th ASM General Meeting (May 2006) [126] and later published in the issue of 15 January 2008 *Journal of Infectious Diseases* [81].

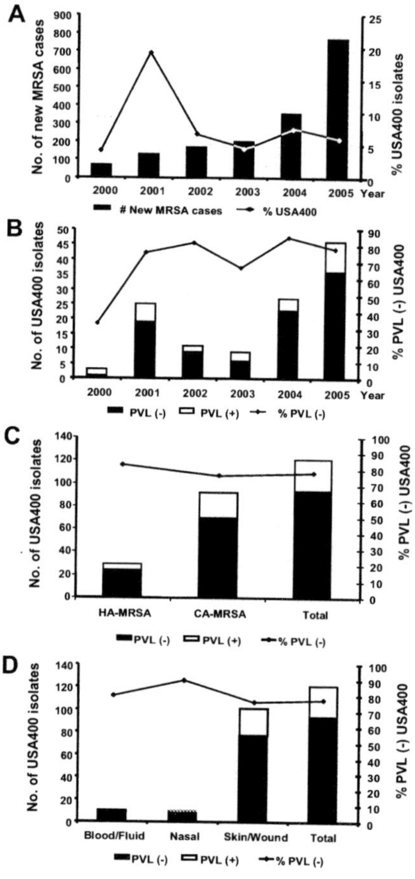

Figure 3. Epidemiology of PVL(+) and PVL(-) USA400 sibling strains. (A) Gradual increase in the number of newly diagnosed cases of MRSA infection/colonization in the Calgary Health Region with stable yearly proportion of USA400 isolates beginning after 2001. (B) Varying yearly number of USA400 isolates with stable proportion of PVL(+)/(-) strains and PVL(-) predominance beginning after 2000. C) USA400 strains were more often associated with infections identified in the community (CA-MRSA) than in the hospital (HA-MRSA) ($p<0.0001$) but with similar PVL carriage rates ($p=0.615$). D) USA400 strains were more often associated with skin/wound infections versus infections of other body sites (blood/sterile fluids and nares) ($p<0.0001$) but with similar PVL carriage rates in isolates from different sources ($p=0.5981$). (Adapted from Zhang et al. 2008 [81].)

Table 1. Toxin, adhesin and exoenzyme virulence gene profiles of PVL(+) and PVL(-) USA400 strains

PFGE profile[b]	No. Isolate	SCC*mec* type[b]	*agr* type[b]	*spa* type[b]	MLST type[b]	Toxin Genes [a]											Adhesin Genes [a]											Exoenzyme Genes [a]		
						sea	seb	sec	sed	see	seg	seh	sei	sej	tst	hlg	fnbA	fnbB	cnaA	cnaB	sdrC	sdrD	sdrE	bbp	ebpS	map/eap	clfA	ica	coa	V8
PVL (-) USA400 (B)	7	IVa	III	t128	ST1	+	-	+	-	-	-	+	-	-	-	+	+	-	+	-	+	+	+	-	+	+	+	+	+	+
PVL (+) USA400 (B)	1	IVa	III	Unamed	ST1	+	-	+	-	-	-	+	-	-	-	+	+	-	+	-	+	+	+	-	+	+	+	+	+	+
PVL (-) USA400 (A)	85	IVa	III	t128	ST1	+	-	+	-	-	-	+	-	-	-	+	+	-	+	-	+	+	+	-	+	+	+	+	+	+
PVL (+) USA400 (A)	26	IVa	III	t128	ST1	+	-	+	-	-	-	+	-	-	-	+	+	-	-	-	+	+	+	-	+	+	+	+	+	+
CMRSA-7	1	IVa	III	t128	ST1	+	-	+	-	-	-	+	-	-	-	+	+	-	-	-	+	+	+	-	+	+	+	+	+	+

Note.

[a] The presence or absence of 25 virulence genes was determined by PCR amplification with previously described primer pairs as indicated in bracket for each gene. Toxin genes: *sea/b/d/e/g/h/i/j*, staphylococcal enterotoxin A/B/C/D/E/G/H/I/J (*sea* [131], *seb/c/d/e* [132], *seg/h/i* [133], *sej* [134]); *tst*, toxic shock syndrome toxin [132]; *hlg*, gamma toxin [96]. Adhesin genes: *fnbA*, fibronectin adhesive molecule A [135]; *fnbB*, fibronectin adhesive molecule B [136]; *cnaA/B*, collagen adhesive molecule A/B [137]; *sdrC/D/E*, putative adhesin [121]; *bbp*, bone sialoprotien adhesin [121]; *ebpS*, elastin adhesin [121]; *map/eap*, major histocompatibility complex class II analogue protein [121]; *clfA*, clumping factor [138]. Exoenzyme genes: *ica*, Polysaccharide intercellular adhesin [121]; *coa*, coagulase [139]; *V8*, Serine protease [121]; *agr* type: accessory gene regulator [121].

[b] PFGE, pulsed field gel electrophoresis; FVL, Panton-Valentine leukocidin; SCC*mec*, staphylococcal cassette chromosome *mec*; *agr*, accessory gene regulator; *spa*, staphylococcal protein A gene (unnamed *spa* type motif: UJJJJJFE); MLST, multilocus sequence typing; +, positive; -, negative.

(Adapted from Zhang et al. 2008 [81].)

Table 2. Clinical features of hospital patients colonized/infected with PVL(+)/(-) USA400 strains [a]

Strain	No	CA/HA-MRSA[b]		Sex		Age of Patient (yrs)				Clinical Feature [c]			
		CA-	HA-	M	F	0-5	6-17	18-65	>65	Colonization	Mild infection	Severe infection	Un-known
PVL(+)	10 (23.8)	7 (36.8)	3 (13.0)	5 (20.0)	5 (29.4)	2 (66.7)	0 (0)	8 (25.8)	0 (0)	1 (8.3)	4 (22.2)	4 (40.0)	1 (50.0)
PVL(-)	32 (76.2)	12 (63.2)	20 (70.0)	20 (80.0)	12 (70.6)	1 (33.3)	3 (100)	23 (74.2)	5 (100)	11 (91.7)	14 (77.8)	6 (60.0)	1 (50.0)
Total	42 (100)	19 (45.2)	23 (54.8)	25 (59.5)	17 (40.5)	3 (7.1)	3 (7.1)	31 (73.8)	5 (11.9)	12 (28.6)	18 (42.9)	10 (23.8)	2 (4.8)

Note.

[a] No. of case with percent in their category in bracket.

[b] CA-MRSA, community-associated methicillin-resistant *Staphylococcus aureus*; HA-MRSA, hospital-associated MRSA.

[c] Refer to the section of Materials and Methods for detailed classification scheme

(Adapted from Zhang et al. 2008 [81].)

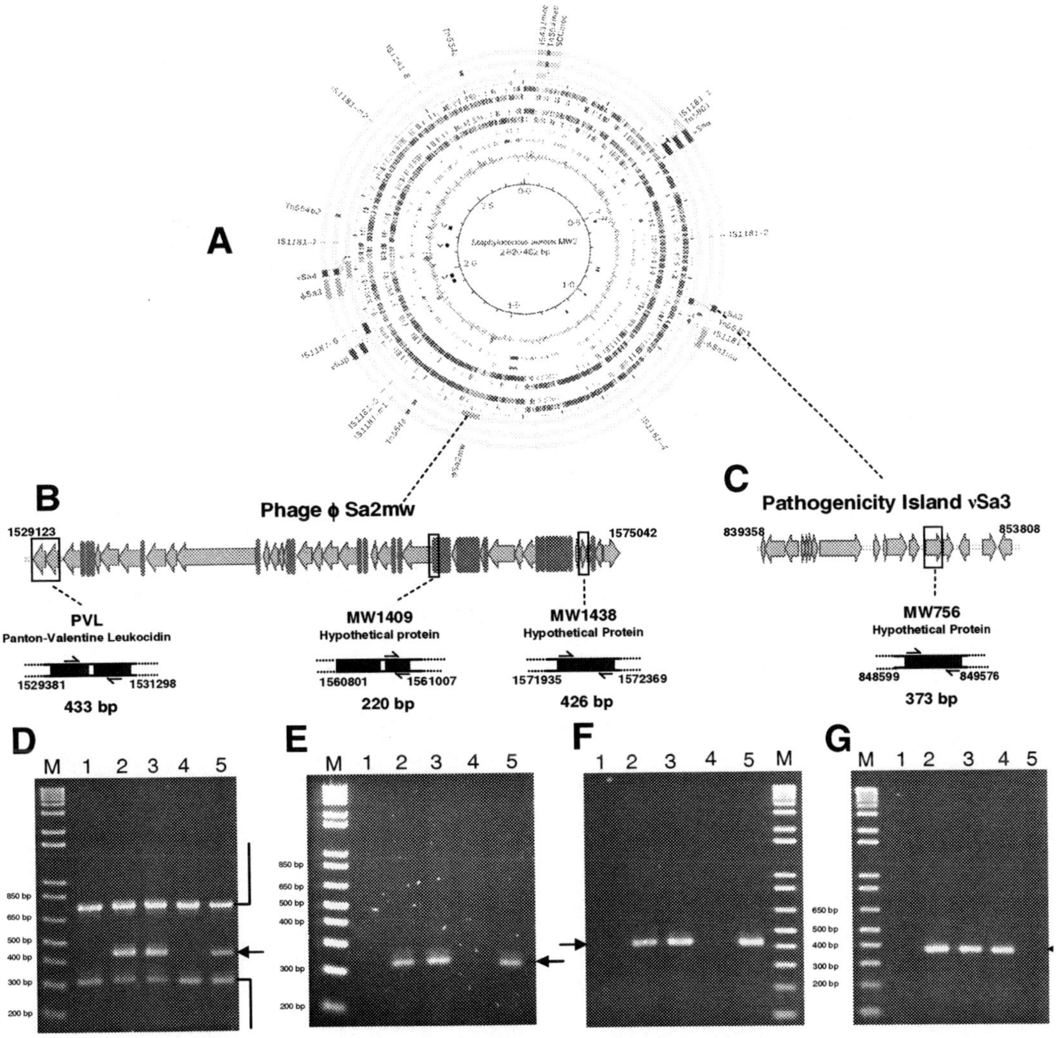

Figure 4. Prophage ϕSa2mw (carrying PVL genes) is present in PVL(+) but absent in PVL(-) USA400 isolates. Depiction of the genome of CA-MRSA USA400 MW2 strain (Reprinted and adapted with permission from Elsevier [91]) (A), the structures of prophage ϕSa2mw (B) and of the pathogenicity island νSa3 (C) with the numbers overlying the genomic sequences delineating the beginning and end of each gene locus. Primers targeting PVL genes and the regions unique to prophage ϕSa2mw (MW1409 and MW1438) and USA400 strain (MW756 in νSa3) are indicated with the genomic sequence number marked and PCR product size (bp) shown. Multiplex PCR (for PVL genes from [97]) and single target PCR (for other unique regions) from the representative isolates are shown in D (PVL genes), E (MW1409), F (MW1438), G (MW756) with an arrow indicating the corresponding PCR product. Lane 1, PVL (-) Canadian epidemic HA-MRSA control strain CMRSA2; lane 2, PVL (+) USA400 control strain CMRSA7; lane 3, PVL (+) USA400 clinical isolate; lane 4, PVL (-) USA400 clinical isolate; lane 5, PVL (+) Canadian epidemic CA-MRSA USA300 control strain CMRSA10; lane M, 1 Kb Plus DNA Ladder (Invitrogen); 16S rRNA, Staphylococcus genus specific 16S rRNA gene primers; *mecA*, methicillin resistance gene. (Adapted from Zhang et al. 2008 [81].)

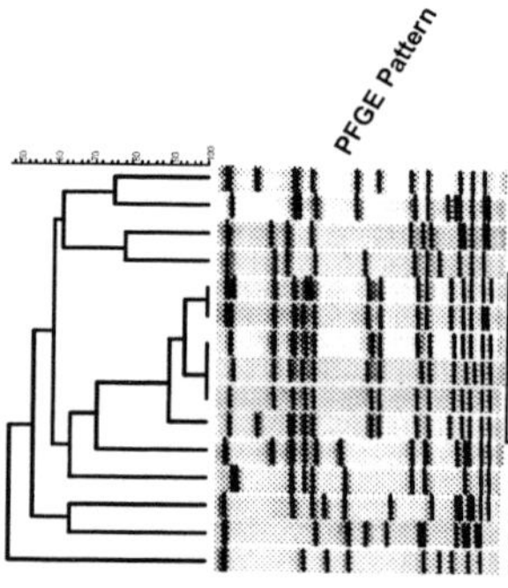

Strain / Isolate	PFGE Profile	No. Isolates	PVL	SCCmec type	agr type	spa type	MLST type	Pen	Oxa	Ery	Clin	Gen	Cip	Tet	Rif	SXT	Van
								Resistance Phenotypes									
CMRSA-5	USA500	1	-	IVd	I	t064	ST8	R	R	R	R	R	R	R	S	R	S
CMRSA-9	NA	1	-	NT	I	t008	ST8	R	R	R	R	R	R	S	S	S	S
CMRSA-3	NA	1	-	III	I	t037	ST241	R	R	R	R	S	R	R	S	R	S
CMRSA-6	NA	1	-	III	I	t037	ST239	R	R	R	R	R	R	R	S	R	S
Isolate	USA400 (B)	7	-	IVa	III	t128	ST1	R	R	R(85.7%)	S	S	S	S	S	S	S
Isolate	USA400 (B)	1	+	IVa	III	Unnamed	ST1	R	R	S	S	S	S	R	S	S	S
Isolate	USA400 (A)	85	-	IVa	III	t128	ST1	R	R	R(82.4%)	S	S	S	R(1.2%)	S	S	S
Isolate	USA400 (A)	26	+	IVa	III	t128	ST1	R	R	R(38.5%)	S	S	S	R(7.7%)	S	S	S
CMRSA-7	USA400 (A)	1	+	IVa	III	t128	ST1	R	R	S	S	S	S	S	S	S	S
Isolate	USA400 (C)	2	-	IVa	III	t128	ST1	R	R	S	S	S	S	S	S	S	S
CMRSA-10	USA300	1	+	IVa	I	t008	ST8	R	R	R	S	S	S	S	S	S	S
CMRSA-2	USA100/800	1	-	II	II	t002	ST5	R	R	R	R	S	R	S	S	S	S
CMRSA-1	USA600	1	-	II	I	t004	ST45	R	R	R	R	R	R	S	S	R	S
CMRSA-8	EMRSA15	1	-	IV	I	t022	ST22	R	R	S	S	S	R	S	S	S	S
CMRSA-4	USA200	1	-	II	III	t018	ST36	R	R	R	S	S	R	S	S	S	S

Figure 5. Shared genotypic and phenotypic traits of PVL(+) and PVL(-) USA400 isolates. Only a single representative isolate from individual pulsed field gel electrophoresis (PFGE) clonotypes is shown. The solid box delineates the groups of USA400 strains with minor PFGE variations (patterns A, B, C as indicated in brackets). CMRSA1-10, Canadian major epidemic MRSA reference strains 1 to 10; Isolate, local clinical isolates of USA400 strains collected in this study; PVL, Panton-Valentine leukocidin (+, positive; -, negative); SCC*mec*, staphylococcal cassette chromosome *mec* (NT: not typeable; ND, not done); *agr*, accessory gene regulator; *spa* (staphylococcal protein A gene) motif: t128 (UJJFKBPE), t002 (TJMBMDMGMK), t004 (A2AKEEMBKB), t008 (YHGFMBQBLO), t018 (WGKAKAOMQQQ), t022 (TJEJNF2MNF2MOMOKR), t037 (WGKAOMQ), t064 (YHGCMBQBLO), Unnamed (UJJJJJFE); MLST (multilocus sequence typing) profile: ST1 (1-1-1-1-1-1-1), ST5 (1-4-1-4-12-1-10), ST8 (3-3-1-1-4-4-3), ST22 (7-6-1-5-8-8-6), ST36 (2-2-2-2-3-3-2), ST45 (10-14-8-6-10-3-2), ST239 (2-3-1-1-4-4-3), ST241 (2-3-1-1-4-4-30); Pen, penicillin; Oxa, Oxacillin; Ery, Erythromycin; Clin, Clindamycin; Gen, Gentamicin; Cip, Ciprofloxacin; Tet, Tetracycline; Rif, Rifampin; Van, Vancomycin; S, susceptible; R, resistant (with resistant rate in brackets). (Adapted from Zhang et al. 2008 [81].)

PVL (+)/(-) CA-MRSA USA400 Sibling Strains Exhibit Similar Virulence Characteristics in *In Vitro* Cell Culture and Animal Models

In order to better understand the role of PVL in virulence and pathogenesis of these PVL-positive and PVL–negative CA-MRSA USA400 sibling strains, we conducted further experimental studies, using various *in vitro* cell culture and animal models to test the virulence properties and characteristics of these sibling strains [127].

The human laryngeal carcinoma cell line HEp-2 was used to study bacterial invasion and survival ability in human cells, by quantifying CFU of intracellular bacteria through serial dilution and plating; while the human lung epithelial cell line A549 was employed to test bacterial cytotoxicity and assayed by reading the OD of solublized Giemsa staining. However, no difference was observed in human laryngeal carcinoma cell invasion/survival ability (Figure 6) and in human lung epithelial cell cytotoxicity (Figure 7) between the PVL (+) and PVL (-) strains (p>0.05), respectively [127].

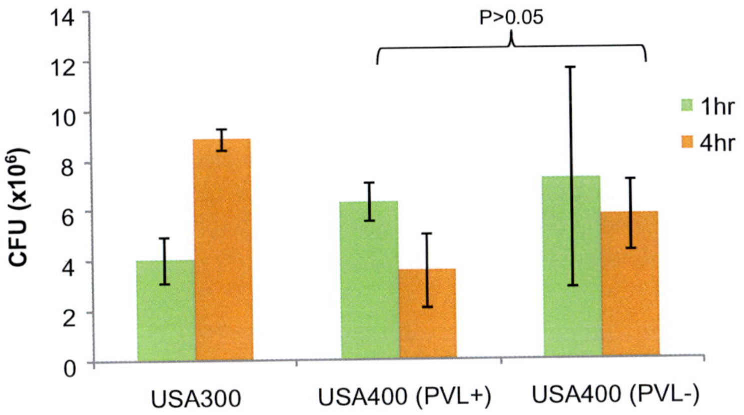

Figure 6. Both PVL(+) and PVL(-) USA400 sibling strains showed similar invasion and survival ability in human laryngeal carcinoma (HEp-2) cells. HEp-2 invasion assay was conduct as follows. 10^5 of HEp-2 cells were seeded into 24-well tissue culture plates about 16hr prior to invasion experiments. S. aureus (~10^8 CFU) were inoculated into each well of HEp-2 cells and incubated for 1hr. The extracellular bacteria were removed by gentamicin and lysostaphin. The intracellular bacteria at 1hr and 4hr were numerated by serial dilution and plating. (Adapted from Wu et al. 2008 [127].)

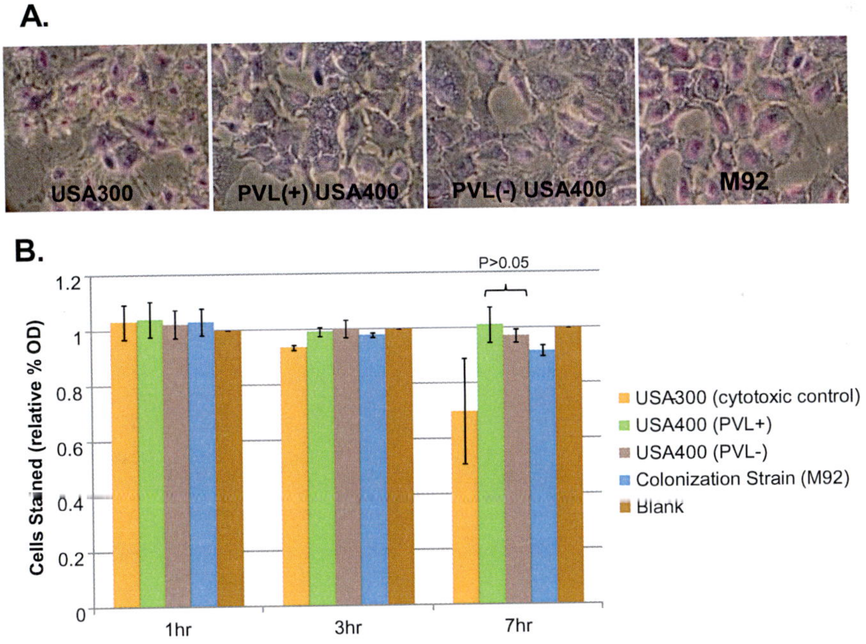

Figure 7. Both PVL(+) and PVL(-) USA400 sibling strains showed no cytotoxicity in human lung epithelial (A549) cells. A549 cell cytotoxicity assay was conducted by seeding 10^5 of A549 cells into 24-well tissue culture plates about 16hr prior to invasion experiments. *S. aureus* (~10^8 CFU) were inoculated into each well of A549 cells and incubated for 1hr. The extracellular bacteria were removed by gentamicin and lysostaphin. At 1hr, 3hr, and 7hr, the cells were fixed with methanol and stained with Giemsa (A). The cytotoxicity was determined by reading the OD of solublized Giemsa staining and expressed as % OD relative to the no-bacterial infection blank control (B). (Adapted from Wu et al. 2008 [127].)

We recently developed and used the nematode *Caenorhabditis elegans* [128] and the fruit fly *Drosophila melanogaster* [129] as host models for studying *S. aureus* virulence and pathogenesis. Three clinical isolates with detailed phenotypic and genotypic characterization from each group of PVL (+) and PVL (-) USA400 sibling strains, plus the USA400 MW2 PVL (+)/(-) isogenic (PVL knockout) strains were selected for testing in these models. Repeatedly, both PVL (+) and PVL (-) USA400 strains showed high nematocidal activity by virtue of killing a majority (>90%) of the nematodes over nine days, with no significant difference in killing rate between these two groups (p>0.05) (Figure 8). The USA400 sibling strains also exhibited a high fly-killing activity in our *Drosophila* model, with more than 85% of flies dead within 60 hours of infection, and no significant difference in killing rates between PVL (+) versus PVL (-) strains (p>0.05) (Figure 9) [127].

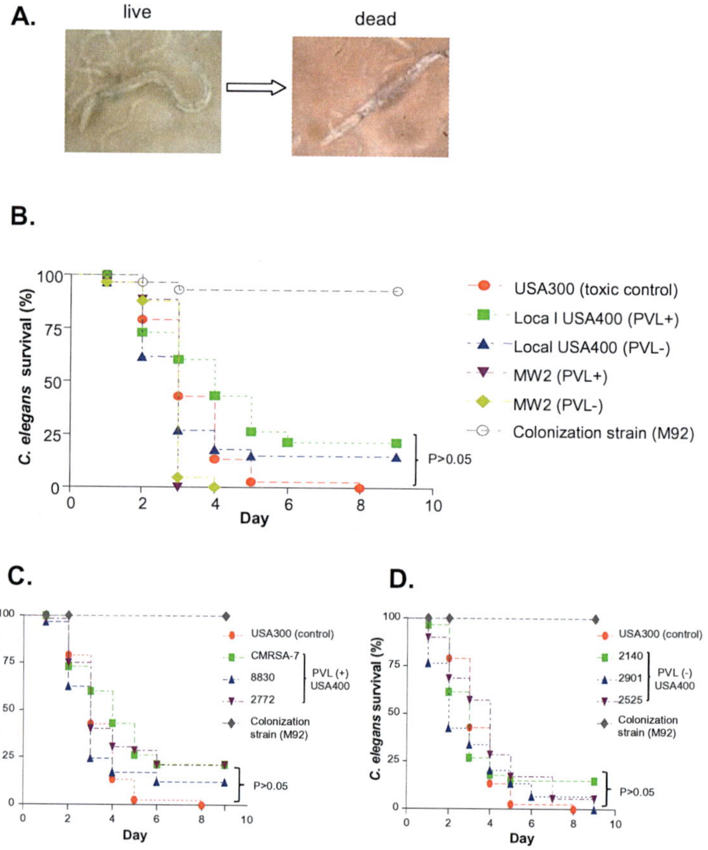

Figure 8. USA400 PVL(+)/(-) sibling strains, similar to control strains (USA400 MW2 and MW2 PVL-knockout) exhibited high nematocidal activities in the *Caenorhabditis elegans* model. Bacteria grown on tryptic soy agar (TSA) plates supplemented with 5µg/ml nalidixic acid (NAL), followed by addition of 30 L4-stage nematodes to each plate, incubation at 25°C, and scoring for live and dead worms every 24 hrs. Experiments were performed in triplicate and repeated at least 3 times. Nematode survival data were analyzed by Kaplan-Meier and log rank tests. Representative images of live and dead *C. elegans* feeding on PVL+ USA400 strain (A). Kaplan-Meier survival plots of nematodes fed PVL(+) and PVL(-) USA400 and control strains (B). Three clinical isolates with detailed phenotypic and genotypic characterization from each group of PVL(+) (C) and PVL(-) (D) USA400 sibling strains demonstrated similar nematode-killing activity. (Adapted from Wu et al. 2008 [127].)

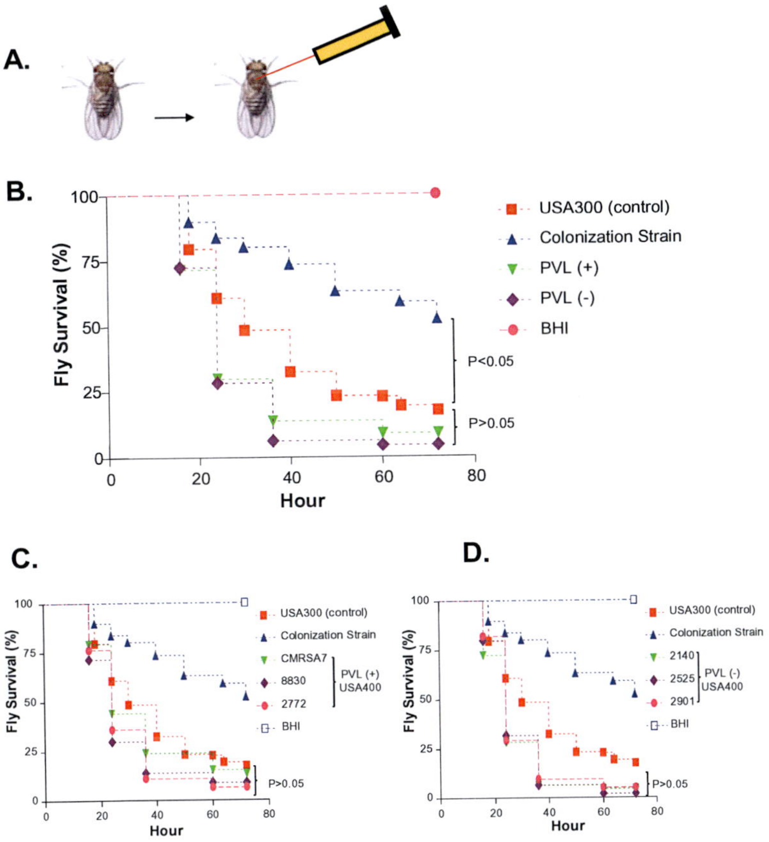

Figure 9. Both PVL(+) and PVL(-) USA400 sibling strains high fly-killing activities in the *Drosophila melanogaster* model. For *Drosophila* killing assay, female flies (2-5 days old) were anesthetized on ice and injected in the dorsal thorax with a 27 gauge needle dipped directly into 200 ml of *S. aureus* bacterial suspension (approximately 8×10^8 CFU/ml) (A). The infected flies were transferred to a vial with sucrose as food supply. The flies were monitored at room temperature and scored as live or dead. Experiments were performed in triplicate and repeated at least 3 times. Fly survival data were analyzed by Kaplan-Meier and log rank tests. Kaplan-Meier survival plots of flies injected with PVL(+) and PVL(-) USA400 and control strains (B). Three clinical isolates with detailed phenotypic and genotypic characterization from each group of PVL(+) (C) and PVL(-) (D) USA400 sibling strains demonstrated similar fly-killing activity. (Adapted from Wu et al. 2008 [127].)

We recently established a murine model capable of demonstrating dermatopathological differences between USA300 and other CA-MRSA strains model [130]. Therefore, we also tested these PVL (+) and PVL (-) USA400 sibling strains in this mouse skin model. Intradermally-induced murine infections caused by both PVL (+) and PVL (-) USA400 sibling strains always identically presented with localized cutaneous infections associated with a focal inflammatory response and no skin ulceration. No dermatopathological difference between these sibling strains was observed. In contrast, infections caused by USA300-positive control strain uniformly presented as extensive open lesions with a histologically-documented profound neutrophilic inflammatory response extending below the fascia, although all mice demonstrated evidence of wound healing after a 14-day period (Figure 10).

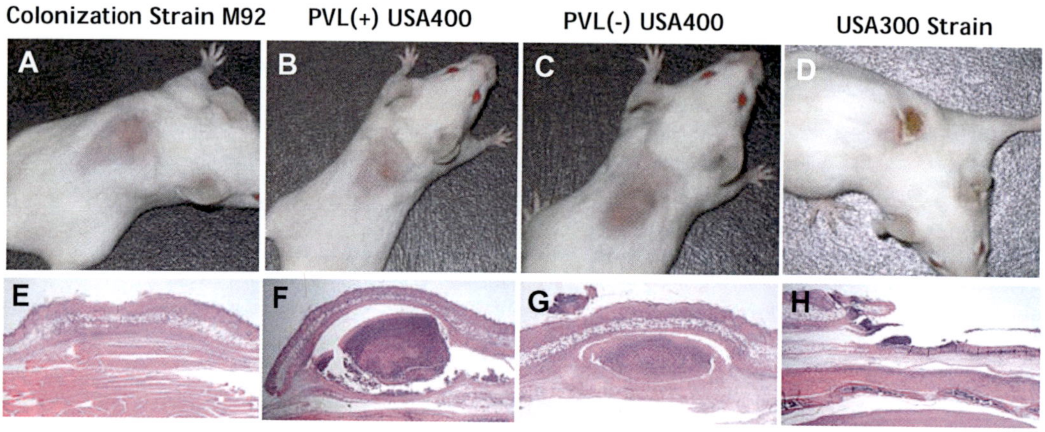

Figure 10. No dermatopathological difference between PVL-positive and -negative sibling strains in a murine intradermal infection model (Day 4). Skin lesions (A-D) and histopathological sections of mouse skin (E-F) from the intradermally infected BABL/c mice. Both PVL(+) (B and F) and PVL(-) (C and G) USA400 sibling strains caused alike pustule/abscess with confined dermal abscess damage without ulceration, in contrast to large cutaneous ulcer with a predominantly neutrophilic inflammation caused by USA 300 strain (D and H) and the localized edema with localized inflammatory reaction without ulceration by colonization strain M92 (A and E). (Adapted from Zhang et al. 2007 [130].)

Our study once more demonstrates that the PVL genes are not the major virulence factor associated with the invasion/cytotoxicity and pathogenesis in various *in vitro* cell culture and animal models, respectively, suggesting that other virulence factors may play a greater role in this regard [127].

Conclusion

The worldwide emergence of CA-MRSA strains has been linked to carriage of PVL genes, although compelling epidemiological data alone are insufficient to establish whether PVL directly contributes to hyper-virulence and widespread dissemination of CA-MRSA infections. The specific role of PVL in the epidemiology and pathogenesis of CA-MRSA infections remains undefined and controversial. Combined with data from murine models, the weight of the evidence currently suggests that the genomic milieu rather than the PVL genes plays the most significant role in the virulence and widespread dissemination of CA-MRSA strains.

Acknowledgment

I am grateful to Dr. John Conly, University of Calgary, for critical review of the manuscript.

References

[1] Lowy, FD. Staphylococcus aureus infections. *N Engl J Med*, 1998, 339(8), 520-32.

[2] Livermore, DM. Antibiotic resistance in staphylococci. *Int J Antimicrob Agents*, 2000, 16 Suppl, 1, S3-10.

[3] Diekema, DJ; Pfaller, MA; Schmitz, FJ; Smayevsky, J; Bell, J; Jones, RN; et al. Survey of infections due to Staphylococcus species: frequency of occurrence and antimicrobial susceptibility of isolates collected in the United States, Canada, Latin America, Europe, and the Western Pacific region for the SENTRY Antimicrobial Surveillance Program, 1997-1999. *Clin Infect Dis*, 2001, 32(Suppl 2), S114-32.

[4] Karchmer, AW. Nosocomial bloodstream infections: organisms, risk factors, and implications. *Clin Infect Dis*, 2000, 31(Suppl 4), S139-43.

[5] Jevons, MP. Celbenin-resistant staphylococci. *British Medical Journal*, 1961, 1, 124-125.

[6] Barber, M. Methicillin-resistant staphylococci. *J Clin Pathol*, 1961, 14, 385-93.

[7] Ito, T; Katayama, Y; Asada, K; Mori, N; Tsutsumimoto, K; Tiensasitorn, C; et al. Structural comparison of three types of staphylococcal cassette chromosome mec integrated in the chromosome in methicillin-resistant *Staphylococcus aureus*. *Antimicrob Agents Chemother*, 2001, 45(5), 1323-36.

[8] Ma, XX; Ito, T; Tiensasitorn, C; Jamklang, M; Chongtrakool, P; Boyle-Vavra, S; et al. Novel type of staphylococcal cassette chromosome mec identified in community-acquired methicillin-resistant Staphylococcus aureus strains. *Antimicrob Agents Chemother*, 2002, 46(4), 1147-52.

[9] Ito, T; Ma, XX; Takeuchi, F; Okuma, K; Yuzawa, H; Hiramatsu, K. Novel type V staphylococcal cassette chromosome mec driven by a novel cassette chromosome recombinase, ccrC. *Antimicrob Agents Chemother*, 2004, 48(7), 2637-51.

[10] Oliveira, DC; Milheirico, C; de Lencastre, H. Redefining a structural variant of staphylococcal cassette chromosome mec, SCCmec type VI. *Antimicrob Agents Chemother*, 2006, 50(10), 3457-9.

[11] Berglund, C; Ito, T; Ikeda, M; Ma, XX; Soderquist, B; Hiramatsu, K. Novel type of staphylococcal cassette chromosome mec in a methicillin-resistant *Staphylococcus aureus* strain isolated in Sweden. *Antimicrob Agents Chemother*, 2008, 52(10), 3512-6.

[12] Zhang, K; McClure, JA; Elsayed, S; Conly, JM. Novel Staphylococcal Cassette Chromosome mec Type Carrying Class A mec and Type 4 ccr Gene Complexes in a Canadian Epidemic Strain of Methicillin-Resistant Staphylococcus aureus *Antimicrob Agents Chemother*, 2008.

[13] Hackbarth, CJ; Chambers, HF. Methicillin-resistant staphylococci: detection methods and treatment of infections Antimicrob. *Agents Chemother*; 1989, 33(7), 995-9.

[14] Hiramatsu, K; Cui, L; Kuroda, M; Ito, T. The emergence and evolution of methicillin-resistant *Staphylococcus aureus*. *Trends Microbiol*, 2001, 9(10), 486-93.

[15] Said-Salim, B; Mathema, B; Kreiswirth, BN. Community-acquired methicillin-resistant *Staphylococcus aureus*: an emerging pathogen. *Infect Control Hosp Epidemiol, 2003*, 24(6), 451-5.

[16] Crossley, K; Loesch, D; Landesman, B; Mead, K; Chern, M; Strate, R. An outbreak of infections caused by strains of *Staphylococcus aureus* resistant to methicillin and aminoglycosides. I. Clinical studies. *J Infect Dis.,* 1979, 139(3), 273-9.

[17] Panlilio, AL; Culver, DH; Gaynes, RP; Banerjee, S; Henderson, TS; Tolson, JS; et al. Methicillin-resistant Staphylococcus aureus in U.S. hospitals, 1975-1991. *Infect Control Hosp Epidemiol*, 1992, 13(10), 582-6.

[18] Voss, A; Milatovic, D; Wallrauch-Schwarz, C; Rosdahl, VT; Braveny, I. Methicillin-resistant *Staphylococcus aureus* in Europe. *Eur J Clin Microbiol Infect Dis.,* 1994, 13(1), 50-5.

[19] Ayliffe, GA. The progressive intercontinental spread of methicillin-resistant *Staphylococcus aureus*. *Clin Infect Dis*., 1997, 24(Suppl 1), S74-9.

[20] Aires de Sousa, M; de Lencastre, H. Bridges from hospitals to the laboratory: genetic portraits of methicillin-resistant *Staphylococcus aureus clones*. *FEMS Immunol Med Microbiol*, 2004, 40(2), 101-11.

[21] Enright, MC; Robinson, DA; Randle, G; Feil, EJ; Grundmann, H; Spratt, BG. The evolutionary history of methicillin-resistant *Staphylococcus aureus* (MRSA). *Proc Natl Acad Sci.,* U S A 2002, 99(11), 7687-92.

[22] Oliveira, DC; Tomasz, A; de Lencastre, H. Secrets of success of a human pathogen: molecular evolution of pandemic clones of methicillin-resistant *Staphylococcus aureus*. *Lancet Infect Dis.,* 2002, 2(3), 180-9.

[23] Deurenberg, RH; Stobberingh, EE. The evolution of Staphylococcus aureus. *Infect Genet Evol*., 2008, 8(6), 747-63.

[24] Udo, EE; Grubb, WB. Genetic analysis of methicillin-resistant *S*taphylococcus aureus from a Nigerian hospital. *J Med Microbiol*, 1993, 38(3), 203-8.

[25] Prevention. CfDCa. Four pediatric deaths from community-acquired methicillin-resistant *Staphylococcus aureus*-Minnesota and North Dakota. 1997-1999. *JAMA*., 1999, 282(12), 1123-5.

[26] Herold, BC; Immergluck, LC; Maranan, MC; Lauderdale, DS; Gaskin, RE; Boyle-Vavra, S; et al. Community-acquired methicillin-resistant *Staphylococcus aureus* in children with no identified predisposing risk. *JAMA*., 1998, 279(8), 593-8.

[27] Vandenesch, F; Naimi, T; Enright, MC; Lina, G; Nimmo, GR; Heffernan, H; et al. Community-acquired methicillin-resistant *Staphylococcus aureus* carrying Panton-Valentine leukocidin genes: worldwide emergence. *Emerg Infect Dis*., 2003, 9(8), 978-84.

[28] Begier, EM; Frenette, K; Barrett, NL; Mshar, P; Petit, S; Boxrud, DJ; et al. A high-morbidity outbreak of methicillin-resistant *Staphylococcus aureus* among players on a college football team, facilitated by cosmetic body shaving and turf burns. *Clin Infect Dis*., 2004, 39(10), 1446-53.

[29] Beilman, GJ; Sandifer, G; Skarda, D; Jensen, B; McAllister, S; Killgore, G; et al. Emerging infections with community-associated methicillin-resistant *Staphylococcus aureus* in outpatients at an Army Community Hospital. *Surg Infect*, (Larchmt) 2005, 6(1), 87-92.

[30] Said-Salim, B; Mathema, B; Braughton, K; Davis, S; Sinsimer, D; Eisner, W; et al. Differential distribution and expression of Panton-Valentine leucocidin among community-acquired methicillin-resistant *Staphylococcus aureus* strains. *J Clin Microbiol*, 2005, 43(7), 3373-9.

[31] Vourli, S; Perimeni, D; Makri, A; Polemis, M; Voyiatzi, A; Vatopoulos, A. Community acquired MRSA infections in a paediatric population in Greece. *Euro Surveill*; 2005, 10(5), 78-9.

[32] Wannet, WJ; Spalburg, E; Heck, ME; Pluister, GN; Willems, RJ; De Neeling, AJ. Widespread dissemination in the Netherlands of the epidemic berlin methicillin-resistant *Staphylococcus aureus* clone with low-level resistance to oxacillin. *J Clin Microbiol*, 2004, 42(7), 3077-82.

[33] Wannet, WJ; Spalburg, E; Heck, ME; Pluister, GN; Tiemersma, E; Willems, RJ; et al. Emergence of virulent methicillin-resistant *Staphylococcus aureus* strains carrying Panton-Valentine leucocidin genes in the Netherlands. *J Clin Microbiol*, 2005, 43(7), 3341-5.

[34] Issartel, B; Tristan, A; Lechevallier, S; Bruyere, F; Lina, G; Garin, B; et al. Frequent carriage of Panton-Valentine leucocidin genes by *Staphylococcus aureus* isolates from surgically drained abscesses. *J Clin Microbiol*, 2005, 43(7), 3203-7.

[35] Robert, J; Etienne, J; Bertrand, X. Methicillin-resistant *Staphylococcus aureus* producing Panton-Valentine leukocidin in a retrospective case series from 12 French hospital laboratories, 2000-2003. *Clin Microbiol Infect*, 2005, 11(7), 585-7.

[36] Ma, XX; Galiana, A; Pedreira, W; Mowszowicz, M; Christophersen, I; Machiavello, S, et al. Community-acquired methicillin-resistant *Staphylococcus aureus*, Uruguay. *Emerg Infect Dis.,* 2005, 11(6), 973-6.

[37] Harbarth, S; Francois, P; Shrenzel, J; Fankhauser-Rodriguez, C; Hugonnet, S; Koessler, T; et al. Community-associated methicillin-resistant *Staphylococcus aureus*, Switzerland. *Emerg Infect Dis.*, 2005, 11(6), 962-5.

[38] Witte, W; Braulke, C; Cuny, C; Strommenger, B; Werner, G; Heuck, D; et al. Emergence of methicillin-resistant *Staphylococcus aureus* with Panton-Valentine leukocidin genes in central Europe. *Eur J Clin Microbiol Infect Dis.*, 2005, 24(1), 1-5.

[39] Holmes, A; Ganner, M; McGuane, S; Pitt, TL; Cookson, BD; Kearns, AM. *Staphylococcus aureus* isolates carrying Panton-Valentine leucocidin genes in England and Wales: frequency, characterization, and association with clinical disease. *J Clin Microbiol*, 2005, 43(5), 2384-90.

[40] Gilbert, M; Gregson, D; Gillespie, J; MacDonald, J; Louie, T; Laupland, K; et al. Clinical Features of Community-Acquired Methicillin-Resistant *S. aureus* (CAMRSA) Skin and Soft Tissue Infections (SSTI) in an Outbreak in Persons with Histories of Drug Use, Homelessness or Incarceration. In: AMMI (Association of Medical Microbiology and Infectious Diseases) Canada-CACMID (Canadian Association for Clinical Microbiology and Infectious Diseases) 2005 Annual Conference, 2005, Ottawa, Ontaria, Canada: *Canadian Journal of Infectious Diseases & Medical Microbiology*, 2005, p. 109.

[41] Mulvey, MR; MacDougall, L; Cholin, B; Horsman, G; Fidyk, M; Woods, S. Community-associated methicillin-resistant *Staphylococcus aureus*, Canada. *Emerg Infect Dis.*, 2005, 11(6), 844-50.

[42] Wylie, JL; Nowicki, DL. Molecular epidemiology of community- and health care-associated methicillin-resistant *Staphylococcus aureus* in Manitoba, Canada. *J Clin Microbiol*, 2005, 43(6), 2830-6.

[43] Gilbert, M; MacDonald, J; Gregson, D; Siushansian, J; Zhang, K; Elsayed, S; et al. Outbreak in Alberta of community-acquired (USA300) methicillin-resistant

Staphylococcus aureus in people with a history of drug use, homelessness or incarceration. *Cmaj.*, 2006, 175(2), 149-54.

[44] Klevens, RM; Morrison, MA; Nadle, J; Petit, S; Gershman, K; Ray, S; et al. Invasive methicillin-resistant *Staphylococcus aureus* infections in the United States. *JAMA.*, 2007, 298(15), 1763-71.

[45] Hota, B; Ellenbogen, C; Hayden, MK; Aroutcheva, A; Rice, TW; Weinstein, RA. Community-associated methicillin-resistant *Staphylococcus aureus* skin and soft tissue infections at a public hospital: do public housing and incarceration amplify transmission? *Arch Intern Med.*, 2007, 167(10), 1026-33.

[46] Larsen, A; Stegger, M; Goering, R; Sorum, M; Skov, R. Emergence and dissemination of the methicillin resistant *Staphylococcus aureus* USA300 clone in Denmark (2000-2005). *Euro Surveill,* 2007, 12(2).

[47] Zetola, N; Francis, JS; Nuermberger, EL; Bishai, WR. Community-acquired meticillin-resistant *Staphylococcus aureus*: an emerging threat. *Lancet Infect Dis.,* 2005, 5(5), 275-86.

[48] Chambers, HF. Community-associated MRSA—resistance and virulence converge. *N Engl J Med.*, 2005, 352(14), 1485-7.

[49] Moran, GJ; Krishnadasan, A; Gorwitz, RJ; Fosheim, GE; McDougal, LK; Carey, RB; et al. Methicillin-resistant *S. aureus* infections among patients in the emergency department. *N Engl J Med.*, 2006, 355(7), 666-74.

[50] Saiman, L; O'Keefe, M; Graham, PL; 3rd Wu, F; Said-Salim, B; Kreiswirth, B; et al. Hospital transmission of community-acquired methicillin-resistant *Staphylococcus aureus* among postpartum women. *Clin Infect Dis.*, 2003, 37(10), 1313-9. Epub 2003, Oct 17.

[51] Perdreau-Remington, F; Carleton, H; Etorma, J; Diep, B; Sensabaugh, G. Alarming prevalence of community-acquired methicilliin resistant *Staphylococcus aureus* (CA-MRSA) in hospitalized patients. In: 44th *Interscience Conference on Antimicrobial Agents and Chemotherapy*, 2004, Washington, DC, USA, 2004.

[52] Healy, CM; Hulten, KG; Palazzi, DL; Campbell, JR; Baker, CJ. Emergence of new strains of methicillin-resistant *Staphylococcus aureus* in a neonatal intensive care unit. *Clin Infect Dis.*, 2004, 39(10), 1460-6.

[53] Bratu, S; Eramo, A; Kopec, R; Coughlin, E; Ghitan, M; Yost, R; et al. Community-associated methicillin-resistant *Staphylococcus aureus* in hospital nursery and maternity units. *Emerg Infect Dis.*, 2005, 11(6), 808-13.

[54] Chalumeau, M; Bidet, P; Lina, G; Mokhtari, M; Andre, MC; Gendrel, D; et al. Transmission of Panton-Valentine leukocidin-producing *Staphylococcus aureus* to a physician during resuscitation of a child. *Clin Infect Dis.*, 2005, 41(3), e29-30.

[55] Linde, H; Wagenlehner, F; Strommenger, B; Drubel, I; Tanzer, J; Reischl, U; et al. Healthcare-associated outbreaks and community-acquired infections due to MRSA carrying the Panton-Valentine leucocidin gene in southeastern Germany. *Eur J Clin Microbiol Infect Dis.*, 2005, 24(6), 419-22.

[56] Naas, T; Fortineau, N; Spicq, C; Robert, J; Jarlier, V; Nordmann, P. Three-year survey of community-acquired methicillin-resistant *Staphylococcus aureus* producing Panton-Valentine leukocidin in a French university hospital. *J Hosp Infect*, 2005.

[57] Klevens, RM; Morrison, MA; Fridkin, SK; Reingold, A; Petit, S; Gershman, K; et al. Community-associated methicillin-resistant *Staphylococcus aureus* and healthcare risk factors. *Emerg Infect Dis.*, 2006, 12(12), 1991-3.

[58] Liu, C; Graber, CJ; Karr, M; Diep, BA; Basuino, L; Schwartz, BS; et al. A population-based study of the incidence and molecular epidemiology of methicillin-resistant *Staphylococcus aureus* disease in San Francisco, 2004-2005. *Clin Infect Dis.*, 2008, 46(11), 1637-46.

[59] Tattevin, P; Diep, BA; Jula, M; Perdreau-Remington, F. Long-term follow-up of methicillin-resistant *Staphylococcus aureus* molecular epidemiology after emergence of clone USA300 in San Francisco jail populations. *J Clin Microbiol*, 2008, 46(12), 4056-7.

[60] Diep, BA; Chambers, HF; Graber, CJ; Szumowski, JD; Miller, LG; Han, LL; et al. Emergence of multidrug-resistant, community-associated, methicillin-resistant *Staphylococcus aureus* clone USA300 in men who have sex with men. *Ann Intern Med.*, 2008, 148(4), 249-57.

[61] Naimi, TS; LeDell, KH; Como-Sabetti, K; Borchardt, SM; Boxrud, DJ; Etienne, J; et al. Comparison of community- and health care-associated methicillin-resistant *Staphylococcus aureus* infection. *JAMA*, 2003, 290(22), 2976-84.

[62] Diep, BA; Otto, M. The role of virulence determinants in community-associated MRSA pathogenesis. *Trends Microbiol*, 2008, 16(8), 361-9.

[63] O'Brien, FG; Lim, TT; Chong, FN; Coombs, GW; Enright, MC; Robinson, DA; et al. Diversity among community isolates of methicillin-resistant *Staphylococcus aureus* in Australia. *J Clin Microbiol*, 2004, 42(7), 3185-90.

[64] Robinson, DA; Kearns, AM; Holmes, A; Morrison, D; Grundmann, H; Edwards G; et al. Re-emergence of early pandemic *Staphylococcus aureus* as a community-acquired methicillin-resistant clone. *Lancet*, 2005, 365(9466), 1256-8.

[65] King, MD; Humphrey, BJ; Wang, YF; Kourbatova, EV; Ray, SM; Blumberg, HM. Emergence of community-acquired methicillin-resistant *Staphylococcus aureus* USA 300 clone as the predominant cause of skin and soft-tissue infections. *Ann Intern Med.*, 2006, 144(5), 309-17.

[66] Zhang, K; McClure, JA; Elsayed, S; Louie, T; Conly, JM. Novel multiplex PCR assay for characterization and concomitant subtyping of staphylococcal cassette chromosome mec types I to V in methicillin-resistant *Staphylococcus aureus*. *J Clin Microbiol*, 2005, 43(10), 5026-33.

[67] Etienne, J. Panton-Valentine leukocidin: a marker of severity for *Staphylococcus aureus* infection? *Clin Infect Dis.*, 2005, 41(5), 591-3.

[68] Voyich, JM; Otto, M; Mathema, B; Braughton, KR; Whitney, AR; Welty, D; et al. Is Panton-Valentine leukocidin the major virulence determinant in community-associated methicillin-resistant *Staphylococcus aureus* disease? *J Infect Dis.*, 2006, 194(12), 1761-70.

[69] Labandeira-Rey, M; Couzon, F; Boisset, S; Brown, EL; Bes, M; Benito, Y; et al. Staphylococcus aureus Panton-Valentine leukocidin causes necrotizing pneumonia. *Science*, 2007, 315(5815), 1130-3.

[70] Bubeck Wardenburg, J; Bae, T; Otto, M; Deleo, FR; Schneewind, O. Poring over pores: alpha-hemolysin and Panton-Valentine leukocidin in *Staphylococcus aureus* pneumonia. *Nat Med.*, 2007, 13(12), 1405-6.

[71] Bubeck Wardenburg, J; Palazzolo-Balance, AM; Otto, M; Schneewind, O; DeLeo, FR. Panton-Valentine leukocidin is not a virulence determinant in murine models of community-associated methicillin-resistant *Staphylococcus aureus* disease. *J Infect Dis.*, 2008, 198(8), 1166-70.

[72] Diep, BA; Palazzolo-Balance, AM; Tattevin, P; Basuino, L; Braughton, KR; Whitney, AR; et al. Contribution of Panton-Valentine leukocidin in community-associated methicillin-resistant *Staphylococcus aureus* pathogenesis. *PLoS ONE*, 2008, 3(9), e3198.

[73] Kernodle, DS. Re: is Panton-Valentine leukocidin the major virulence determinant in community-associated methicillin-resistant *Staphylococcus aureus* disease? *J Infect Dis.*, 2007, 195(11), 1726, author reply 1727-8.

[74] Schwartzman, WA; Beenhouwer, DO; Schaberg, DR. How relevant were the models used to measure the impact of Panton-Valentine leukocidin in human staphylococcal infections? *J Infect Dis.*, 2007, 195(11), 1726-7, author reply 1727-8.

[75] Grojec, PL; Jeljaszewicz, J. Effect of staphylococcal leukocidin on mouse leukocyte system. *Zentralbl Bakteriol Mikrobiol Hyg.*, [A] 1981, 250(4), 446-55.

[76] Rittirsch, D; Hoesel, LM; Ward, PA. The disconnect between animal models of sepsis and human sepsis. *J Leukoc Biol.*, 2007, 81(1), 137-43.

[77] Zhang, K; McClure, J; Lau, V; Elsayed, S; Hutchins, W; Louie, T; et al. Genetic Diversity Among Panton-Valentine Leukocidin (PVL)+ *Staphylococcus aureus* Isolates over 16 Years: Lack of Evidence to Support PVL as a Major Determinant Associated with the Emergence of Community-Associated MRSA (C-MRSA). *In: 45th Interscience Conference on Antimicrobial Agents and Chemotherapy*, 2005 December, 16 - 19, 2005, Washington, DC, USA, 2005.

[78] Diep, BA; Carleton, HA; Chang, RF; Sensabaugh, GF; Perdreau-Remington, F. Roles of 34 virulence genes in the evolution of hospital- and community-associated strains of methicillin-resistant *Staphylococcus aureus*. *J Infect Dis.*, 2006, 193(11), 1495-503.

[79] Rossney, AS; Shore, AC; Morgan, PM; Fitzgibbon, MM; O'Connell, B; Coleman, DC. The emergence and importation of diverse genotypes of methicillin-resistant *Staphylococcus aureus* (MRSA) harboring the Panton-Valentine leukocidin gene (pvl) reveal that pvl is a poor marker for community-acquired MRSA strains in Ireland. *J Clin Microbiol*, 2007, 45(8), 2554-63.

[80] Monecke, S; Slickers, P; Ellington, MJ; Kearns, AM; Ehricht, R. High diversity of Panton-Valentine leukocidin-positive, methicillin-susceptible isolates of *Staphylococcus aureus* and implications for the evolution of community-associated methicillin-resistant *S. aureus*. *Clin Microbiol Infect*, 2007, 13(12), 1157-64.

[81] Zhang, K; McClure, JA; Elsayed, S; Tan, J; Conly, JM. Coexistence of Panton-Valentine leukocidin-positive and -negative community-associated methicillin-resistant *Staphylococcus aureus* USA400 sibling strains in a large Canadian health-care region. *J Infect Dis.*, 2008, 197(2), 195-204.

[82] van de Velde, H. Etude sur le me´canisme de la virulence du Staphylocoque pyoge`ne. *La Cellule*, 1894, 10, 401-60.

[83] Panton, PN; Valentine, FCO. Staphylococcal toxin. *Lancet*, 1932, 222, 506-508.

[84] Finck-Barbancon, V; Prevost, G; Piemont, Y. Improved purification of leukocidin from *Staphylococcus aureus* and toxin distribution among hospital strains. *Res Microbiol*, 1991, 142(1), 75-85.

[85] Woodin, AM. Purification of the two components of leucocidin from *Staphylococcus aureus*. *Biochem J*, 1960, 75, 158-65.

[86] Noda, M; Kato, I. Purification and crystallization of staphylococcal leukocidin. *Methods Enzymol*, 1988, 165, 22-32.

[87] Kaneko, J; Kamio, Y. Bacterial two-component and hetero-heptameric pore-forming cytolytic toxins: structures, pore-forming mechanism, and organization of the genes. *Biosci Biotechnol Biochem*, 2004, 68(5), 981-1003.

[88] Prevost, G; Cribier, B; Couppie, P; Petiau, P; Supersac, G; Finck-Barbancon, V; et al. Panton-Valentine leucocidin and gamma-hemolysin from Staphylococcus aureus ATCC 49775 are encoded by distinct genetic loci and have different biological activities. *Infect Immun.*, 1995, 63(10), 4121-9.

[89] Kaneko, J; Kimura, T; Narita, S; Tomita, T; Kamio, Y. Complete nucleotide sequence and molecular characterization of the temperate staphylococcal bacteriophage phiPVL carrying Panton-Valentine leukocidin genes. *Gene.*, 1998, 215(1), 57-67.

[90] Narita, S; Kaneko, J; Chiba, J; Piemont, Y; Jarraud, S; Etienne, J; et al. Phage conversion of Panton-Valentine leukocidin in Staphylococcus aureus: molecular analysis of a PVL-converting phage, phiSLT. *Gene.*, 2001, 268(1-2), 195-206.

[91] Baba, T; Takeuchi, F; Kuroda, M; Yuzawa, H; Aoki, K; Oguchi, A; et al. Genome and virulence determinants of high virulence community-acquired MRSA. *Lancet*, 2002, 359(9320), 1819-27.

[92] Ma, XX; Ito, T; Chongtrakool, P; Hiramatsu, K. Predominance of clones carrying Panton-Valentine leukocidin genes among methicillin-resistant *Staphylococcus aureus* strains isolated in Japanese hospitals from 1979 to 1985. *J Clin Microbiol*, 2006, 44(12), 4515-27.

[93] Ma, XX; Ito, T; Kondo, Y; Cho, M; Yoshizawa, Y; Kaneko, J; et al. Two different Panton-Valentine leukocidin phage lineages predominate in Japan. *J Clin Microbiol*, 2008, 46(10), 3246-58.

[94] Deurenberg, RH; Vink, C; Driessen, C; Bes, M; London, N; Etienne, J; et al. Rapid detection of Panton-Valentine leukocidin from clinical isolates of *Staphylococcus aureus* strains by real-time PCR. *FEMS Microbiol Lett.*, 2004, 240(2), 225-8.

[95] Johnsson, D; Molling, P; Stralin, K; Soderquist, B. Detection of Panton-Valentine leukocidin gene in *Staphylococcus aureus* by LightCycler PCR: clinical and epidemiological aspects. *Clin Microbiol Infect*, 2004, 10(10), 884-9.

[96] Lina, G; Piemont, Y; Godail-Gamot, F; Bes, M; Peter, MO; Gauduchon, V; et al. Involvement of Panton-Valentine leukocidin-producing *Staphylococcus aureus* in primary skin infections and pneumonia. *Clin Infect Dis.*, 1999, 29(5), 1128-32.

[97] McClure, JA; Conly, JM; Lau, V; Elsayed, S; Louie, T; Hutchins, W; et al. Novel multiplex PCR assay for detection of the staphylococcal virulence marker Panton-Valentine leukocidin genes and simultaneous discrimination of methicillin-susceptible from -resistant staphylococci. *J Clin Microbiol*, 2006, 44(3), 1141-4.

[98] McDonald, RR; Antonishyn, NA; Hansen, T; Snook, LA; Nagle, E; Mulvey, MR; et al. Development of a Triplex Real-Time PCR Assay for Detection of Panton-Valentine Leukocidin Toxin Genes in Clinical Isolates of Methicillin-Resistant *Staphylococcus aureus*. *J Clin Microbiol*, 2005, 43(12), 6147-6149.

[99] Nakagawa, S, Taneike, I; Mimura, D; Iwakura, N; Nakayama, T; Emura, T; et al. Gene sequences and specific detection for Panton-Valentine leukocidin. *Biochem Biophys Res Commun*, 2005, 328(4), 995-1002.

[100] Supersac, G; Prevost, G; Piemont, Y. Sequencing of leucocidin R from *Staphylococcus aureus* P83 suggests that staphylococcal leucocidins and gamma-hemolysin are members of a single, two-component family of toxins. *Infect Immun*, 1993, 61(2), 580-7.

[101] Pedelacq, JD; Maveyraud, L; Prevost, G; Baba-Moussa, L; Gonzalez, A; Courcelle, E; et al. The structure of a *Staphylococcus aureus* leucocidin component (LukF-PV) reveals the fold of the water-soluble species of a family of transmembrane pore-forming toxins. *Structure Fold Des.*, 1999, 7(3), 277-87.

[102] Prevost, G; Bouakham, T; Piemont, Y; Monteil, H. Characterisation of a synergohymenotropic toxin produced by *Staphylococcus intermedius. FEBS Lett.*; 1995, 376(3), 135-40.

[103] Menestrina, G; Serra, MD; Prevost, G. Mode of action of beta-barrel pore-forming toxins of the staphylococcal alpha-hemolysin family. *Toxicon*, 2001, 39(11), 1661-72.

[104] Prevost, G; Couppie, P; Prevost, P; Gayet, S; Petiau, P; Cribier, B; et al. Epidemiological data on *Staphylococcus aureus* strains producing synergohymenotropic toxins. *J Med Microbiol*, 1995, 42(4), 237-45.

[105] Ward, PD; Turner, WH. Identification of staphylococcal Panton-Valentine leukocidin as a potent dermonecrotic toxin. *Infect Immun.*, 1980, 28(2), 393-7.

[106] Woodin, AM. Staphylococcal leukocidin. In: Montje TC, editor. *Microbial Toxins.* Burlington, MA, USA: *Academic Press Inc.*, 1970, p. 327-355.

[107] Gillet, Y; Issartel, B; Vanhems, P; Fournet, JC; Lina, G; Bes, M; et al. Association between *Staphylococcus aureus* strains carrying gene for Panton-Valentine leukocidin and highly lethal necrotising pneumonia in young immunocompetent patients. *Lancet*, 2002, 359(9308), 753-9.

[108] Gonzalez, BE; Martinez-Aguilar, G; Hulten, KG; Hammerman, WA; Coss-Bu, J; Avalos-Mishaan, A; et al. Severe Staphylococcal sepsis in adolescents in the era of community-acquired methicillin-resistant *Staphylococcus aureus. Pediatrics*, 2005, 115(3), 642-8.

[109] Miller, LG; Perdreau-Remington, F; Rieg, G; Mehdi, S; Perlroth, J; Bayer, AS; et al. Necrotizing fasciitis caused by community-associated methicillin-resistant *Staphylococcus aureus* in Los Angeles. *N Engl J Med.*, 2005, 352(14), 1445-53.

[110] Francis, JS; Doherty, MC; Lopatin, U; Johnston, CP; Sinha, G, Ross, T; et al. Severe community-onset pneumonia in healthy adults caused by methicillin-resistant *Staphylococcus aureus* carrying the Panton-Valentine leukocidin genes. *Clin Infect Dis.*, 2005, 40(1), 100-7.

[111] Klein, JL; Petrovic, Z; Treacher, D; Edgeworth, J. Severe community-acquired pneumonia caused by Panton-Valentine leukocidin-positive *Staphylococcus aureus*: first reported case in the United Kingdom. *Intensive Care Med.*, 2003, 29(8), 1399. Epub 2003 May 29.

[112] Miyashita, T; Shimamoto, Y; Nishiya, H; Koshibu, Y; Sugiyama, H; Ono Y, et al. Destructive pulmonary embolism in a patient with community-acquired staphylococcal bacteremia. *J Infect Chemother*, 2002, 8(1), 99-102.

[113] Reichert, B; Birrell, G; Bignardi, G. Severe non-pneumonic necrotising infections in children caused by Panton-Valentine leukocidin producing *Staphylococcus aureus* strains. *J Infect*; 2005, 50(5), 438-42.

[114] Peleg, AY; Munckhof, WJ; Kleinschmidt, SL; Stephens, AJ; Huygens, F. Life-threatening community-acquired methicillin-resistant *Staphylococcus aureus* infection in Australia. *Eur J Clin Microbiol Infect Dis.*, 2005, 24(6), 384-7.

[115] Tseng, MH; Wei, BH; Lin, WJ; Lu, JJ, Lee, SY; Wang, SR; et al. Fatal sepsis and necrotizing pneumonia in a child due to community-acquired methicillin-resistant *Staphylococcus aureus*: case report and literature review. *Scand J Infect Dis.*, 2005, 37(6-7), 504-7.

[116] Adem, PV; Montgomery, CP; Husain, AN; Koogler, TK; Arangelovich, V, Humilier M, et al. *Staphylococcus aureus* sepsis and the Waterhouse-Friderichsen syndrome in children. *N Engl J Med.*, 2005, 353(12), 1245-51.

[117] Cribier, B; Prevost, G; Couppie, P; Finck-Barbancon, V; Grosshans, E; Piemont, Y. *Staphylococcus aureus* leukocidin: a new virulence factor in cutaneous infections? An epidemiological and experimental study. *Dermatology*, 1992, 185(3), 175-80.

[118] Mulvey, MR; Chui, L; Ismail, J; Louie, L; Murphy, C; Chang, N; et al. Development of a Canadian standardized protocol for subtyping methicillin-resistant *Staphylococcus aureus* using pulsed-field gel electrophoresis. *J Clin Microbiol*, 2001, 39(10), 3481-5.

[119] Enright, MC; Day, NP; Davies, CE; Peacock, SJ; Spratt, BG. Multilocus sequence typing for characterization of methicillin-resistant and methicillin-susceptible clones of *Staphylococcus aureus*. *J Clin Microbiol*, 2000, 38(3), 1008-15.

[120] Harmsen, D; Claus, H; Witte, W; Rothganger, J; Turnwald, D; Vogel, U. Typing of methicillin-resistant *Staphylococcus aureus* in a university hospital setting by using novel software for spa repeat determination and database management. *J Clin Microbiol*, 2003, 41(12), 5442-8.

[121] Peacock, SJ; Moore, CE; Justice, A; Kantzanou, M; Story, L; Mackie, K; et al. Virulent combinations of adhesin and toxin genes in natural populations of *Staphylococcus aureus*. *Infect Immun*, 2002, 70(9), 4987-96.

[122] Feil, EJ; Li, BC; Aanensen, DM; Hanage, WP; Spratt, BG. eBURST: inferring patterns of evolutionary descent among clusters of related bacterial genotypes from multilocus sequence typing data. *J Bacteriol*; 2004, 186(5), 1518-30.

[123] Spratt, BG; Hanage, WP; Li, B; Aanensen, DM; Feil, EJ. Displaying the relatedness among isolates of bacterial species the eBURST approach *FEMS Microbiol Lett.*, 2004, 241(2), 129-34.

[124] Tomita, Y; Kawano, O; Ichiyasu, H; Fukushima, T; Fukuda, K; Sugimoto, M; et al. [Two cases of severe necrotizing pneumonia caused by community-acquired methicillin-resistant *Staphylococcus aureus*]. *Nihon Kokyuki Gakkai Zasshi*, 2008, 46(5), 395-403.

[125] Jungk, J; Como-Sabetti, K; Stinchfield, P; Ackerman, P; Harriman, K. Epidemiology of methicillin-resistant *Staphylococcus aureus* at a pediatric healthcare system, 1991-2003. *Pediatr Infect Dis., J* 2007, 26(4), 339-44.

[126] Zhang, K; McClure, J; Tan, J; Elsayed, S; Conly, J. Co-Existence of Panton-Valentine Leukocidin (PVL)-Positive and -Negative Sibling Community-Associated MRSA (C-MRSA) USA400 Strains with Identical Molecular and Phenotypic Characteristics in a

Large Canadian Healthcare Region. In: the 106th General Meeting of American Society for Microbiology, 2006, *Orlando*, *Florida*, *USA*, 2006.

[127] Wu, K; Conly, J; McClure, J; Elsayed, S; Zhang, K. Panton-Valentine Leukocidin (PVL)-Positive and -Negative Community-Associated MRSA (CA-MRSA) USA400 Sibling Strains Exhibit Similar Virulence Characteristics in In Vitro Cell Culture and Animal Models. In: the 13th International Symposium on Staphylococci & Staphylococcal Infections. *Cairns*, *Australia*, 2008.

[128] Wu, K; Conly, J; McClure, J; Elsayed, S; Louie, T; Zhang, K. Caenorhabditis elegans as a Host Model for Community-Associated Methicillin-Resistant *Staphylococcus aureus*. *Clinical Microbiology and Infection*, 2008, (in press).

[129] Wu, K; Conly, J; McClure, J; Surette, M; Sibley, C; Elsayed, S; et al. Drosophila melanogaster as a Host Model for Community-Associated Methicillin-Resistant *Staphylococcus aureus* (CA-MRSA). In: The 13th International Symposium on Staphylococci & Staphylococcal Infections. *Cairns*, *Australia*, 2008.

[130] Zhang, K; Armstrong, G; McClure, J; Mulvey, G; Barber, D; Hyland, R; et al. A Murine Model Capable of Demonstrating Dermatopathological Differences between High-Transmissibility (USA300) and Hypervirulent (USA400) Strains of Community-Associated MRSA (CA-MRSA). In: the Association of Medical Microbiology & Infectious Disease Canada (AMMI Canada)-Canadian Association for Clinical Microbiology & Infectious Diseases (CACMID) 2007 Annual Conference. *Halifax*, *Nova Scotia*, *Canada*, 2007.

[131] Tsen, HY; Chen, TR. Use of the polymerase chain reaction for specific detection of type A, D and E enterotoxigenic *Staphylococcus aureus* in foods. *Appl Microbiol Biotechnol,* 1992, 37(5), 685-90.

[132] Johnson, WM; Tyler, SD; Ewan, EP; Ashton, FE; Pollard, DR; Rozee, KR. Detection of genes for enterotoxins, exfoliative toxins, and toxic shock syndrome toxin 1 in *Staphylococcus aureus* by the polymerase chain reaction. *J Clin Microbiol*, 1991, 29(3), 426-30.

[133] Jarraud, S; Cozon, G; Vandenesch, F; Bes, M; Etienne, J; Lina, G. Involvement of enterotoxins G and I in staphylococcal toxic shock syndrome and staphylococcal scarlet fever. *J Clin Microbiol*, 1999, 37(8), 2446-9.

[134] Monday, SR; Bohach, GA. Use of multiplex PCR to detect classical and newly described pyrogenic toxin genes in staphylococcal isolates. *J Clin Microbiol*, 1999, 37(10), 3411-4.

[135] Signas, C; Raucci, G; Jonsson, K; Lindgren, PE; Anantharamaiah, GM; Hook, M; et al. Nucleotide sequence of the gene for a fibronectin-binding protein from *Staphylococcus aureus*: use of this peptide sequence in the synthesis of biologically active peptides. *Proc Natl Acad Sci*., U S A 1989, 86(2), 699-703.

[136] Jonsson, K; Signas, C; Muller, HP; Lindberg, M. Two different genes encode fibronectin binding proteins in *Staphylococcus aureus*. The complete nucleotide sequence and characterization of the second gene. *Eur J Biochem*, 1991, 202(3), 1041-8.

[137] Switalski, LM; Patti, JM; Butcher, W; Gristina, AG; Speziale, P; Hook, M. A collagen receptor on Staphylococcus aureus strains isolated from patients with septic arthritis mediates adhesion to cartilage. *Mol Microbiol*, 1993, 7(1), 99-107.

[138] Stephan, R; Annemuller, C; Hassan, AA; Lammler, C. Characterization of enterotoxigenic *Staphylococcus aureus* strains isolated from bovine mastitis in north-east Switzerland. *Vet Microbiol*, 2001, 78(4), 373-82.
[139] Hookey, JV; Richardson, JF; Cookson, BD. Molecular typing of *Staphylococcus aureus* based on PCR restriction fragment length polymorphism and DNA sequence analysis of the coagulase gene. *J Clin Microbiol* 1998;36(4):1083-9.

Reviewed by

Dr. John Conly, University of Calgary and Calgary Health Region, Calgary, Alberta, Canada.

In: Cross Infections: Types, Causes and Prevention
Editors: Jin Dong and Xun Liang

ISBN: 978-1-60741-467-4
© 2009 Nova Science Publishers, Inc.

Chapter III

Catheter-Related Infections: Etiology, Pathogenesis, Diagnosis and Prevention

Maria de Lourdes Ribeiro de Souza da Cunha*
Department of Microbiology and Immunology, Biosciences Institute, São Paulo State University (UNESP), Botucatu, SP, Brazil

Abstract

The advent of intensive care units (ICUs) has led to advances in the treatment of critical-care patients, increasing the survival even of high risk populations such as septic, immunodepressed and oncologic patients and very-low-weight preterm newborns. However, the evolution of the therapeutic arsenal using increasingly more invasive techniques has resulted in the breakdown of barriers and the exposure of previously intact tissues that thus become susceptible to infection. Catheter-related infections (CRI) are one example of this reality and occur when a microorganism invades the bloodstream through a vascular catheter. Infections associated with the use of intravascular devices account for 10 to 20% of all nosocomial infections and are one of the most frequent causes of morbidity and mortality, representing a source of bacteremia and sepsis in hospitalized patients and increasing the length of hospital stay, hospitalization costs and mortality. Approximately 65% of these infections result from the migration of microorganisms of the skin microbiota from the insertion site of the catheter. Intraluminal contamination is observed in 30% of cases and 5% occur through other routes such as infusion of contaminated fluids and distant infectious foci. All of these contamination sources are important, but the most prevalent is contamination with microorganisms of the patient himself in areas close to the insertion site of the catheter. This explains why coagulase-negative staphylococci (CNS) are the microorganisms most frequently associated with this type of infection since they are also the most common in skin. CRI are diagnosed when identical microorganisms are isolated from catheter cultures and

* Corresponding Author: Departamento de Microbiologia e Imunologia, Instituto de Biociências, Universidade Estadual Paulista (UNESP), Botucatu, SP, Brasil. Caixa Postal 510, CEP 18618-000. Tel. 55 (14) 3811-6058 Fax: 55 (14) 3815-3744. E-mail: cunhamlr@ibb.unesp.br

from blood cultures in the absence of any apparent source of infection, except for the catheter. The reliability of catheter cultures for the diagnosis of CRI depends on the culture technique used. The objective of this chapter was to review various aspects of CRI such as diagnosis, incidence, etiology, pathogenesis, main recommended preventive measures, use of catheters impregnated with antiseptic, antimicrobial and anticoagulant agents, and new prevention strategies based on the knowledge of the mechanisms of bacterial adhesion and biofilm formation. Biofilm formation is regulated by the exchange of chemical signals between cells during a process called "quorum-sensing". A new approach to prevent the colonization of catheters and to reduce infections related to these devices is to interfere with this cell-cell communication which permits these microorganisms to organize themselves into complex biofilms, protecting them from the host immune system and conferring greater resistance to antimicrobials.

Introduction

Central vascular catheters (CVC) are indispensable tools in modern medical practice for the care of critical-care patients, especially in intensive care units (ICUs). The use of these devices has resulted in lower mortality even in high-risk populations such as patients with sepsis, immunodepressed patients, cancer patients, and very low birthweight preterm newborns [1]. However, the advances in the therapeutic arsenal using increasingly more invasive techniques have resulted in the breakdown of barriers and the exposure of previously intact tissues which consequently become susceptible to infection. Venous catheters are essential for the care of hospitalized patients who require a central access and their advantages are practically indisputable. However, although CVC permits vascular access necessary for treatment and diagnosis, the use of these devices is associated with risks of local infection and systemic complications, including thrombophlebitis, endocarditis, bacteremia, and sepsis [1, 2].

More than 150 million vascular catheters are implanted annually at hospitals and clinics in the United States. Most of these devices are peripheral venous catheters, but an expressive number (more than 5 million) are CVC inserted into deep or central vessels [3]. More than 200,000 cases of bloodstream infections are reported in the United States, most of them related to non-tunneled CVC. The purpose of these catheters is variable and includes the administration of drugs, blood and blood derivatives, parenteral nutrition, monitoring of the hemodynamic condition of the patient, and vascular access for hemodialysis [4].

Infections associated with the use of intravascular devices account for 10 to 20% of all nosocomial infections and are one of the most frequent causes of morbidity and mortality, representing a source of bacteremia and sepsis in hospitalized patients. The incidence of vascular access infections is lower when compared to infections that occur at other sites (urinary tract: 40-42%, respiratory tract: 11-32%, surgical wound: 8-24%, and bloodstream: 5-9%), but their severity and lethality are higher, exceeding 30% in some cases [5, 6].

The risk factors associated with intravascular catheter-related infections include the duration of catheterization, site of insertion, catheter material, presence of multiple lumen catheters, skin colonization at the insertion site, the microorganisms involved in colonization, frequent manipulation, type of dressing used, underlying disease, and severity of the clinical status of the patient as well as his immunological condition [7, 8].

Central Venous Access Catheters

According to the Centers for Disease Control and Prevention (CDC) [1], the following catheters are used for venous and arterial access:

- Peripheral venous catheter: A short (< 8 cm) catheter usually inserted into peripheral veins of the forearm or hand for short-term venous access, which is rarely associated with bloodstream infection. Phlebitis is observed with prolonged use.
- Peripheral arterial catheter: A short (< 8 cm) catheter generally inserted into the radial arteries or, alternatively, into the femoral, axillary, brachial or posterior tibial artery, presenting a low risk of infection and rarely being associated with bloodstream infection.
- Midline catheter: A catheter (8 to 20 cm) inserted through the antecubital fossa into basilic or cephalic proximal veins that does not enter central veins, i.e., a peripheral catheter. Anaphylactoid reactions have been reported for catheters consisting of hydrogel and elastomer. The rates of phlebitis are lower than those observed for short peripheral catheters.
- Non-tunneled central venous catheter: A catheter inserted percutaneously into central veins (subclavian, internal jugular or femoral vein). It is the most commonly used catheter and is responsible for most catheter-related bloodstream infections (CRBSI). The catheter measures 8 cm in length or more depending on the size of the patient.
- Pulmonary artery catheter: A catheter inserted through a Teflon introducer into a central vein (subclavian, internal jugular or femoral vein). The catheter is generally lined with heparin to reduce the risk of thrombosis and microbial adherence. CRBSI rates are similar to those of CVC. Subclavian insertion is preferred to reduce the risk of infection. The catheter measures 30 cm in length or more depending on the size of the patient.
- Peripherally inserted central venous catheter: A catheter inserted into the basilic, cephalic or brachial veins which enters the superior vena cava. The infection rate is lower than that of non-tunneled CVC. The catheter measures 20 cm in length or more depending on the size of the patient.
- Tunneled central venous catheter: A catheter (Hickman, Broviac, Groshong or Quinton catheter) surgically implanted through a subcutaneous tunnel with placement of a Dacron cuff close to the exit site to inhibit the migration of microorganisms and stimulate the adhesion of underlying tissue sealing the tunnel. This catheter is indicated for patients requiring prolonged vascular access (chemotherapy, home infusion or hemodialysis). The cuff prevents migration of microorganisms into the catheter tract. The infection rate is lower than that observed for non-tunneled CVC. The catheter measures 8 cm in length or more depending on the size of the patient.
- Totally implantable catheter: A surgically implanted catheter which is tunneled below the skin and possesses a subcutaneous port accessed with a needle. The catheter is implanted into the subclavian or internal jugular vein and presents the lowest risk of CRBSI. Catheter site care is not required. Surgery is necessary for removal of the catheter. The catheter measures 8 cm in length or more depending on the size of the patient.

- Umbilical catheter: A catheter inserted in the umbilical vein or artery of newborns during the first days of life. The risk of CRBSI is similar for umbilical vein and artery catheters. The catheter measures 6 cm in length or less depending on the size of the patient.

Incidence of Catheter-Related Infections

Table 1 summarizes the data reported by the National Nosocomial Infection Surveillance System (NNIS) for the period from January 1992 and June 2004 [9] regarding the incidence of catheter-related infections according to the type of ICU.

In neonatal ICUs, the infection rate is inversely proportional to newborn birthweight, ranging from 9.1 per 1000 catheter-days in children with a birthweight <1000 g to 3.5 per 1000 catheter-days in children weighing >2500 g (Table 2).

Most CRBSI are caused by coagulase-negative staphylococci. According to NNIS data [10] covering the period from 1992 to 1999, these microorganisms were responsible for 37% of CRBSI, followed by *Staphylococcus aureus* (13%) and *Enterococcus* (13%). Gram-negative bacteria such as the enterobacteria *Escherichia coli*, *Enterobacter* and *Klebsiella pneumoniae* and the non-fermenting Gram-negative bacilli *Pseudomonas aeruginosa* and *Acinetobacter baumannii* are isolated in about 28% of these infections. *Candida* spp. is the causative agent of about 8% of CRBSI, most of them being non-albicans species including *Candida parapsilosis*, *C. glabrata* and *C. krusei* [1, 10].

Table 1: Incidence of catheter-related infections according to the type of intensive care unit (ICU).

Type of ICU	Mean rate/1000 catheter-days
Coronary	3.5
Medical-Cardiothoracic	2.7
Neurosurgical	4.6
Pediatric	6.6
Surgical	4.6
Trauma	7.4
Burn	7.0
Respiratory	4.8

Source: NNIS [9].

Table 2: Incidence of catheter-related infections among newborns according to birthweight.

Birthweight (g)	Mean rate/1000 catheter-days
≤1000	9.1
1001 - 1500	5.4
1501 - 2500	4.1
>2500	3.5

Source: NNIS [9].

Pathogenesis of Catheter-Related Infections

The pathogenesis of catheter-related infections is complex and only partially understood, with speculations that these infections are directly associated with the adherence of microorganisms that become able to colonize the device. There are four potential sources for catheter colonization and the occurrence of CRBSI: the site of catheter insertion in the skin, catheter hub, hematogenic route and contamination of the infusate. The skin insertion site is the main source of colonization and infection in short-term catheters. Bacteria present on the patient's skin migrate along the outer surface of the catheter to colonize the distal tip and produce infection [11]. Catheter hub colonization is another source of infection. In this case, microorganisms are probably introduced by the hands of the healthcare team, contaminating the hub and migrating along the inner surface of the catheter, thus producing bloodstream infection. Colonization of the inner surface is expected to increase with prolonged use of the catheter hub (more than 30 days) [12]. Hematogenic contamination of CVC from a distant infectious focus, such as pneumonia, gastrointestinal infection or urinary tract infection, has been suggested but is not an important cause of catheter colonization and is rarely confirmed [13]. Various cases of epidemic bacteremia related to contamination of the infusate have been reported [14]. Parenteral nutrition solutions and lipid emulsions promote the growth of many bacteria and fungi such as *Candida parapsilosis* and *Malassezia furfur* [15]. Although many epidemics of nosocomial bacteremia are caused by contaminated infusate, its contribution to endemic primary nosocomial bacteremias is very low.

All routes of catheter contamination are important, but none of them more than contamination by skin microorganisms. Particularly, coagulase-negative staphylococci represent a threat since they are commonly found in the skin microbiota, a fact that explains why they are the microorganisms most frequently isolated from these infections.

Microbial adherence to the catheter surface depends on the interaction between three factors: host, microorganisms and catheter material. The host reacts against the catheter by recognizing it as a foreign body and forms a cover consisting of fibrin and fibronectin around it. These host protein components covering the catheter surface permit the adherence of *S. aureus*. These bacteria produce coagulase which promotes thrombogenesis, as well as various other surface proteins which contain receptors for proteins released by the host such as fibrinogen and fibronectin that permit adherence and colonization of the catheter [16]. Coagulase-negative staphylococci can colonize the native surface of the catheter as well as surfaces conditioned by these host proteins. Once adhered, these bacteria multiply forming multiple layers and producing an extracellular polysaccharide known as slime or biofilm, which potentiates their pathogenicity. The biofilm does not only favor the adherence of microorganisms but also their maintenance by acting as a barrier against attacks by antibiotics, neutrophils, phagocytes, macrophages, and antibodies. The concentration of an antibiotic necessary to destroy bacteria in a biofilm is 100 to 1000 times higher than that required to destroy the same species in suspension, a fact impairing treatment and increasing the possibility of recurrent infections since the bacteria are protected from the host immune system [17].

Candida is also a matter of concern since studies have shown that these species are responsible for about 80% of nosocomial fungal infections. In addition, some species produce a biofilm similar to the bacterial one in the presence of glucose-containing solutions, a fact explaining the increase in the proportion of CRBSI due to fungal pathogens especially among patients receiving parenteral nutrition [18].

The third factor important for microbial adherence is the catheter material. *In vitro* studies have demonstrated that polyvinyl chloride or polyethylene catheters are less resistant to microbial adherence than catheters made of Teflon, silicone or polyurethane [1].

Prevention and Control of Catheter-Related Infections

The length of hospital stay, mortality rates and hospitalization costs increase significantly in patients with CRBSI. This infection prolongs hospitalization by 6.5 to 22 days and adds a cost of US$29,000 to US$56,000 per episode of infection. Mortality is estimated to be 13% to 28% higher in patients with these infections compared to patients sharing the same severity but without this complication [19, 20].

Intensive efforts aimed at the prevention and control of catheter-related infections have been made by local, state and federal agencies, professional societies, universities, research institutes, and national and international organizations. In this respect, evidence-based educational programs, together with strategies reinforcing desired professional behavior, are a valuable tool to be used to modify the attitude of healthcare workers [20]. Europe and the United States occupy a leading position in the application of educational strategies as a facilitating tool to reduce the rates of vascular catheter-related infections. For example, in the United States the 2002 Guidelines published by the CDC [1] for the prevention of CRBSI are recommendations categorized on the basis of existing scientific evidence, i.e., the results of experimental studies, clinical trials or epidemiological studies are used to recommend the implementation of a certain preventive measure (Table 3).

Table 3: Categories according to the CDC [1].

Category	Nature of the study
IA	Strongly recommended for implementation and strongly supported by well-designed experimental, clinical, or epidemiological studies.
IB	Strongly recommended for implementation and supported by some experimental, clinical, or epidemiological studies and a strong theoretical rationale.
IC	Required by state or federal regulations, rules, or standards.
II	Suggested for implementation and supported by suggestive clinical or epidemiological studies or a theoretical rationale.
Unresolved	Practices for which evidence is insufficient or no consensus regarding efficacy exists.

According to the CDC, training and education of the health team including techniques for passage, maintenance care and insertion of vascular catheters are categorized as IA, with the healthcare workers being encouraged to constantly seek updates in the literature and replies to their questions. The care of patients with CVC is performed according to guidelines established in national and international clinical and epidemiological studies and, in certain situations, by the opinion or clinical experience of professionals in that area. The impact of the training of healthcare workers on the incidence of CRBSI has been demonstrated by Yilmaz et al. [21] in a 495-bed teaching hospital, who observed significant improvement (p=0.004) in the CRBSI rate after a period of training. The infection rate was low during the first 3 months of training, but increased 2.08 times after the third month. The authors concluded that regular training of residents who are in charge of inserting catheters and of nurses and interns responsible for catheter maintenance is highly effective in reducing CRBSI rates. Comparison of the incidence of CRBSI between the pre-education and post-education period showed a reduction of 41.7%. A reduction in the incidence of CRBSI by education-based interventions has also been reported by Warren et al. [6], with a decline from 12.9% pre-intervention to 9.4% post-intervention.

With respect to the catheter insertion technique, various recommendations based on IA evidence are available, including aseptic insertion techniques. Procedures such as hand hygiene are fundamental and are always indicated when the healthcare worker comes in contact with the patient. Handwashing should always be performed using soap containing an antiseptic or alcohol gel [1]. Skin antisepsis is fundamental before insertion of the catheter and during dressing change. Although 2% chlorhexidine is preferred, iodine tincture, iodophor or 70% alcohol may also be used [1]. According to some investigators, the presence of microorganisms on the skin around the insertion site is strongly associated with subsequent infection. Despite local antisepsis before insertion of the catheter, bacteria inhabiting this area might be introduced into deeper tissue layers during the procedure [22, 23].

The selection of the catheter, insertion technique and insertion site associated with the lowest risk of complications for the type and duration of intravenous therapy is fundamental. *In vitro* studies have demonstrated that polyvinyl chloride and polyethylene catheters are less resistant to microbial adherence than catheters made of Teflon, silicone or polyurethane [1, 24]. The possibility of microbial adherence to the catheter surface has encouraged manufacturers to fabricate CVC with minimal surface irregularities. The catheter material should be flexible enough to permit free passage through the vasculature but not to such an extent that it would tend to twist or break. In addition, certain materials are more thrombogenic than others, a characteristic also associated with catheter colonization and consequent infection [25].

Also with respect to risk factors, the use of multiple lumen CVC has advantages for patients who require different intravenous medications, laboratory tests, transfusions of blood derivatives and parenteral nutrition. Since their introduction, these catheters have been preferred for patients requiring a central access. However, multiple lumen catheters may result in higher rates of colonization and CRBSI because of their frequent manipulation, with the possible inoculation of microorganisms [26]. The use of CVC with a minimum number of lumens essential for treatment is recommended on the basis CDC evidence IB [1]1.

Regarding the catheter insertion technique, specialists recommend the use of maximum sterile barrier precautions, such as a sterile gown, sterile gloves, sterile sheet, cap and mask, in order to prevent device-associated infections [1, 27].

There are numerous studies in the literature evaluating the antimicrobial activity of antiseptics, demonstrating the efficacy of 2% chlorhexidine gluconate compared to 10% iodine tincture or 70% alcohol. In a meta-analysis of randomized controlled clinical trials, Chaiyakunapruk et al. [28] found a significantly lower incidence of CRBSI in patients who received chlorhexidine gluconate for antisepsis of the insertion site. Young et al. [27]

compared the use of 2% chlorhexidine and 10% povidone-iodine for skin antisepsis during CVC insertion and observed a reduction in the CRBSI rate from 11.3 per 1000 CVC-days to 3.7 per 1000 CVC-days.

With respect to the occurrence of infections at the site of catheter insertion, attention should be paid to the density of the local skin microbiota. Various studies have recommended the preferential insertion of CVC into the subclavian vein. Catheters inserted into the internal jugular vein possess a higher risk of infection because of their proximity to oropharyngeal secretions, in addition to difficulties in fixation necessary to guarantee their immobility [1, 29]. Insertion through the femoral vein should be avoided in view of the elevated risk of complications such as deep venous thrombosis and infection [1, 30]. In addition to professional skills, the choice of the insertion site should also take into account factors inherent to the patient such as anatomical deformities, tracheostomy, mechanical complications and risk of bleeding, among others [1].

The most widely used catheter site dressing materials are semipermeable transparent polyurethane films, followed by dressings using gauze and adhesive tape [1]. The aspects related to these dressings are complex and controversial, with each dressing presenting advantages and disadvantages [31]. Transparent dressings permit visual inspection of the insertion site and changes are less frequent; however, these dressings favor the formation of humidity and are not recommended for patients with intense exudate discharge. In cases of drainage (blood or body fluid) or perspiration, a gauze dressing is preferred [1, 31]. The purpose of the use of dressings in CVC is to reduce extrinsic contamination and local trauma. The dressing should be kept clean and dry in order to permit continuous inspection for the early detection of local complications of intravenous therapy. Dressings should be examined daily and changed if they become wet, dirty or loose [1].

According to the CDC [1], application of topical antibiotics (polymyxin, bacitracin and neomycin) to the catheter insertion site is not recommended. Studies on this subject were unable to show a prophylactic effect. In addition, topical antibiotics may promote fungal infection and antimicrobial resistance.

Removal of the intravascular devices as soon as their use is no longer necessary is recommended according to CDC evidence IA [1]. Catheters and cuffs coated with antimicrobial agents or antiseptics may decrease the risk of CRBSI and potentially reduce hospital costs associated with the treatment of these infections despite the cost of the acquisition of catheters impregnated with antimicrobials/antiseptics [1]. These catheters have been approved by the FDA for use in patients weighing ≥ 3 kg. However, there are currently no antimicrobial-impregnated catheters available for use in children weighing less than 3 kg [1]. Catheters impregnated with chlorhexidine/silver sulfadiazine only on the outer surface have been studied as a tool to reduce CRBSI. Two meta-analyses have demonstrated that these catheters reduce the risk of CRBSI when compared to standard non-impregnated catheters [32, 33]. In another meta-analysis, mean duration of catheterization ranged from 5.1 to 11.2 days [34]. The half-life of *in vitro* antimicrobial activity against *S. epidermidis* is 3 days for catheters impregnated with chlorhexidine/silver sulfadiazine, with this activity declining over time [35].

A second generation of catheters coated with chlorhexidine on the inner and outer surface is now available. The outer surface contains a 3 times higher amount of chlorhexidine and antiseptic release is increased when compared to first-generation catheters. The outer surface of the catheter is coated with chlorhexidine combined with silver sulfadiazine and the inner surface is coated with chlorhexidine alone. Studies indicate that prolonged antimicrobial activity improves the efficacy of protection against infections [36]. Although rare, anaphylaxis has been reported with the use of these chlorhexidine/silver sulfadiazine-impregnated catheters in Japan [37]. However, whether the microorganisms that colonize the catheter and cause infection become resistant to chlorhexidine/silver sulfadiazine has not been established [34].

Chlorhexidine/silver sulfadiazine-impregnated catheters can save costs in the range of US$ 68 to US$391 per catheter in patients at high risk of CRBSI even in the presence of other preventive strategies (e.g., maximum barrier precautions and aseptic techniques). The use of these catheters can be cost-effective in patients hospitalized in ICUs, burn patients, neutropenic patients and other patient populations in which the infection rate exceeds 3.3 per 1000 catheter-days [1, 38]. In a multicenter clinical trial, CVC impregnated on the outer and inner surface with minocycline/rifampicin were associated with lower CRBSI rates when compared to first-generation chlorhexidine/silver sulfadiazine-impregnated catheters [7]. A beneficial effect was observed after day 6 of catheterization but none of the catheters was evaluated beyond 30 days. There was no report of organisms resistant to minocycline/rifampicin. However, *in vitro* data indicate that these impregnated catheters may increase the incidence of minocycline and rifampicin resistance among pathogens, especially staphylococci. The half-life of *in vitro* antimicrobial activity against *S. epidermidis* is 25 days for catheters coated with minocycline/rifampicin compared to 3 days for first-generation chlorhexidine/silver sulfadiazine-impregnated catheters [39]. The duration of *in vivo* antimicrobial activity is also longer for minocycline/rifampicin-coated catheters compared to first-generation chlorhexidine/silver sulfadiazine-impregnated catheters [7].

There are no comparative studies using second-generation chlorhexidine/silver sulfadiazine-impregnated catheters. Studies are necessary to determine whether there is improvement in the antimicrobial activity of catheters coated with minocycline/rifampicin compared to catheters impregnated on the inner and outer surface with chlorhexidine/silver sulfadiazine. As done for chlorhexidine/silver sulfadiazine-impregnated catheters, some clinicians have recommended minocycline/rifampicin-coated catheters for patient populations when the CRBSI rate exceeds 3.3 per 1000 catheter-days [34]. The decision to use chlorhexidine/silver sulfadiazine- or minocycline/rifampicin-impregnated catheters should be based on the decision to improve CRBSI prevention after standard procedures have been implemented (e.g., education of the healthcare team, maximum barrier precautions, and use of 2% chlorhexidine for skin antisepsis), as well as on the concern about the emergence of resistant pathogens and the cost of the implemented strategy [1].

The infusion of anticoagulant substances is widely used for the prevention of catheter thrombosis. Thrombi and fibrin deposits in catheters may promote the adherence of microbial pathogens to the surface and consequent colonization of intravascular catheters, and anticoagulants therefore play a role in the prevention of CRBSI [40]. In a meta-analysis evaluating the benefits of heparin prophylaxis in patients with short-term CVC, the risk of CVC-related thrombosis was found to be reduced with the use of prophylactic heparin [41]. However, no substantial difference in the CRBSI rate was observed. Anticoagulants are mainly administered in the case of long-term catheters in which catheter hub and luminal colonization are causes of CRBSI. Most pulmonary artery, umbilical and central vascular catheters are heparinized [1].

Daily infusion of vancomycin in combination with heparin has been shown to reduce the risk of catheter infection [42]. However, the CDC [1] does not recommend the use of vancomycin as a prophylactic agent for the prevention of CRBSI since it is an independent risk factor for the acquisition of vancomycin-resistant enterococci. In addition, the prolonged use of vancomycin may result in the emergence of staphylococci with intermediate vancomycin resistance.

A new infusion solution containing minocycline and EDTA has been developed [39], which is characterized by broad spectrum and frequent synergistic activity against oxacillin-resistant staphylococci, Gram-negative bacilli and *Candida albicans*. This combination has also proved to be highly effective in a clinical trial for the prevention of staphylococcal infections of long- and short-term catheters [39]. A more recent randomized prospective study demonstrated the efficacy of this combination for the prevention of CRBSI in hemodialysis patients with CVC for long-term access. The combination of minocycline and EDTA presents the same or an even stronger anticoagulant activity than heparin which is not reduced by the addition of minocycline [43, 44]. In addition, these drugs are not used for the treatment of bloodstream infections and, therefore, the risk of occurrence of resistant microorganisms is low. This solution is used to prevent recurrent catheter-related infections in high-risk patients [40].

Diagnosis of Catheter-Related Infections

Until recently, there was no consensus regarding the diagnosis of catheter-related infections. In 2002, the CDC standardized these concepts by differentiating between significant catheter colonization and catheter-related sepsis. According to the CDC [1], significant catheter colonization is characterized by a strong correlation between local catheter inflammation and isolation of more than 15 colony-forming units (CFU) of a microorganism per catheter segment. Therefore, the term "local infection" is frequently employed in this situation. Other investigators use the term "colonization" to describe this event in contrast to the term "contamination" when fewer than 15 CFU are isolated. However, a positive catheter segment culture in the absence of a positive blood culture cannot be considered catheter-related bacteremia or fungemia.

The term sepsis or CRBSI is used when the same microorganism (species and antibiogram) of a semiquantitative culture (≥ 15 CFU per catheter segment) or quantitative culture (≥ 1000 CFU per catheter segment) is isolated by culture of a blood sample from a patient with clinical signs of sepsis (fever, hypothermia, apnea) and no apparent source of infection except for the catheter. Therefore, the definitive diagnosis is established when the catheter is significantly colonized with the same microorganism as found in the blood culture [1]. It should be emphasized that the lack of standard clinical and diagnostic criteria and the diversity of concepts of infection compromise the epidemiological surveillance system of infections and impair generalization of the results of studies.

Within this context, before the development of a semiquantitative culture technique most clinical microbiology laboratories used broth culture of catheter tips for qualitative assessment. This technique resulted in poorly reliable and nonspecific data that did not permit the distinction between colonization and infection. In a recent study comparing qualitative and semiquantitative culture for the diagnosis of CRBSI in newborns, Marconi et al. [45] observed that, despite a lower sensitivity (90%), semiquantitative culture presented higher specificity (71%) than the qualitative technique (100% sensitivity, 60% specificity). The authors concluded that the semiquantitative catheter-tip culture method presented advantages for the diagnosis of CRBSI in newborns when compared to the traditional qualitative method.

The reliability of culture depends on the technique used. The semiquantitative culture method proposed by Maki et al. [46], or roll plate method (catheter rolled over a blood agar plate), is the technique most used for the determination of CRBSI rates. The semiquantitative roll plate culture method is the simplest and most frequently used and its importance has been demonstrated in various studies. Maki et al. [46] showed that semiquantitative catheter-tip culture growing ≥ 15 CFU was better correlated with the presence of infection than qualitative broth culture of the catheter tip in which infection and contamination are indistinguishable. However, these authors found only four cases of catheter-related sepsis, all of them associated with the number of microorganisms with confluent growth. Analyzing these results the authors discussed that the cut-off of ≥ 15 CFU required further evaluation for the determination of the number of CFU that was best correlated with the presence of CRBSI without reducing the sensitivity of the test. Within this context, Marconi et al. [47] determined the cut-off of semiquantitative culture that was best correlated with the presence of CRBSI in newborns. Eighty-five catheter tips from 63 newborns were studied. The microorganisms isolated from the catheters and peripheral blood samples were identified and the drug sensitivity of the isolates was tested by the disk diffusion method. The optimum cut-off was determined using a receiver-operating characteristic (ROC) curve and the definitive diagnosis of CRBSI by isolation of the same microorganism (species and drug sensitivity profile) in catheter culture and peripheral blood cultures, in the absence of any apparent focus of infection except for the catheter, was used as the gold standard. Eight (72.7%) of the 11 episodes of infection diagnosed were associated with coagulase-negative staphylococci, with *S. epidermidis* being identified in six cases. The optimum cut-off for the diagnosis of catheter-related infection defined by the ROC curve was ≥ 122 CFU, with a sensitivity and specificity of 91.0% and 81.1%, respectively, compared to 91.0% sensitivity and 71.6% specificity when a cut-off ≥ 15 CFU was used. Although most cases of CRBSI grew more than 122 CFU, in one case of infection caused by *Staphylococcus aureus* the culture grew only 8 CFU. Cases of CRBSI whose cultures grew < 15 CFU have also been reported by other investigators [5]. These results might be explained by the administration of antibiotics before culture or intraluminal contamination of the catheter, the latter being a limiting factor of the semiquantitative culture method which only detects microorganisms adhered to the outer surface of the device [48]. This technique is rather limited in the case of long-term catheters in which the inner surface is the main source of colonization. This disadvantage is not observed for quantitative techniques such as the vortex or sonication method. The vortex method described by Brun-Buisson et al. [49] consists of flushing the catheter lumen with sterile distilled water to detach microorganisms from the inner surface, followed by serial dilution and seeding onto blood agar plates. Growth ≥ 1000 CFU/ml is indicative of CRBSI.

One disadvantage of these semiquantitative and quantitative culture methods is the need for removal of the catheter for culture. Thus, other diagnostic methods of CRBSI that do not require removal of the device should be considered. The most promising methods are those that permit maintenance of the access. This advantage is particularly important in the case of critical-care patients with difficult vascular access and patients with long-term catheters. This fact has led to the development of new techniques for the diagnosis of CRBSI that do not require catheter removal. One of these new techniques is the differential-time-to-positivity method (DTP) in which qualitative blood samples are collected from the CVC and peripheral vein and microbial growth is monitored continuously. A time interval of positivity between the CVC and peripheral blood cultures of more than 2 hours indicates CRBSI. Thus, if automatic recording of the time of microbial growth in the peripheral and catheter blood cultures reveals a positive result in the catheter culture 2 or more hours before the blood culture, the test is considered to be positive. Another technique is quantitative paired blood culture of samples drawn from the catheter and peripheral vein, in which microbial growth at least 5-fold higher in the catheter culture compared to the peripheral blood culture indicates a positive result [50].

The DTP method is simpler than quantitative blood culture and widely available since many clinical microbiology laboratories have adopted the use of automated systems for blood culture monitoring. Thus, this technique can be used in large prospective clinical trials as an easy and less costly method for the diagnosis of CRBSI that does not require catheter removal [51]. In the study of Blot at al. [51], CRBSI was diagnosed in 16 of 17 patients who presented a positive blood culture of samples collected from the CVC at least 2 hours before the peripheral blood culture, with the test showing 91% sensitivity and 94% specificity.

New Perspectives in the Control of Catheter-Related Infections

According to many investigators, the biofilm is responsible for most bacterial infections and for 65% of vascular catheter-related infections. Biofilm formation is considered to be the result of microbial adherence, the formation of microcolonies and the production of extracellular polysaccharides by these microorganisms. Most CVC become colonized with microorganisms embedded in a biofilm on the surface of the catheter 24 hours after insertion and colonization of the catheter lumen is observed after 8 days. In some cases, the microorganisms will multiply and reach a number sufficient to produce CRBSI. Within this context, the determination of biofilm production by microorganisms isolated from blood cultures drawn from the catheter may contribute to the decision of whether or not to remove the device.

Different methods are currently used for the detection of *Staphylococcus* biofilm, complemented by molecular methods (polymerase chain reaction, PCR) that provide direct evidence of the genetic basis of biofilm production. The simplest available techniques that can be used in clinical laboratory routine are qualitative methods, such as the tube adherence assay proposed by Christensen et al. [52] and the Congo red agar method described by Freeman et al. [53]. The former is the one most commonly used. Various authors have reported reliable results for this method, which was found to be effective, showing excellent sensitivity and adequate specificity and providing a reliable and adequate diagnosis for routine use.

Various regulatory systems are involved in the determination of *S. aureus* virulence, with the best characterized being the *agr* and *sar* systems [54]. The *agr* system consists of two operons that are transcribed in opposite directions. The operon transcribed from P2 encodes the RNAII molecule which regulates the expression of the *agrB*, *agrD*, *agrC* and *agrA* genes. This operon interacts with the *sar* system which controls the transcription of an mRNA, called RNAIII, which regulates the expression of *S. aureus* virulence genes. Genes encoding adhesins are expressed in the logarithmic phase of bacterial growth, whereas in the stationary phase the RNAIII molecule inhibits the expression of these genes and induces the expression of toxin-encoding genes. The *agr* system is controlled by quorum sensing, a signaling system used by bacteria. In the case of high cell density, this system permits bacteria to "feel" the best time for the expression of virulence factors and to guarantee that the combined attack against the host is efficient. The principle of quorum sensing is simple: when a single bacterium secretes an autoinducer into the environment its concentration is too low to be detected; however, when a sufficient number of bacteria are present the concentration of autoinducers reaches an adequate level that permits cells to respond to a stimulus by activating or inhibiting target genes.

A new approach to prevent colonization and biofilm formation by *S. aureus* and *S. epidermidis* is to interfere with the cell-cell communication that results in the virulence phenotype. RNAIII synthesis is regulated by the above mentioned quorum sensing mechanism and can be inhibited with RNAIII-inhibiting peptide (RIP). RIP is a linear peptide produced by coagulase-negative staphylococci (*S. warneri* or *S. xylosus* have been suggested). The peptide consists of a seven amino-acid sequence, YSPXTNF, where X can be a cysteine, tryptophan or a modified amino acid [55-57]. Both natural RIP and a synthetic analog (YSPXTNF) are extremely effective in the inhibition of RNAIII synthesis *in vitro* and *in vivo*. Studies have shown a marked reduction in the pathogenic potential of *S. aureus* when the bacterium is preincubated in the presence of RIP. Various studies using animal models have demonstrated strong activity in terms of the prevention of *S. aureus* infections, including those caused by drug-resistant strains such as methicillin-resistant *S. aureus* and vancomycin-intermediate *S. aureus*. No toxicity was reported and resistant strains have not emerged. RIP inhibits cell-cell communication by interfering with quorum sensing mechanisms, reducing toxin production and adherence properties. Studies investigating the adherence of *S. aureus* to host cells clearly demonstrated that RIP not only reduces the number of adhered bacteria but also adherence properties [56]. Balaban et al. [56] examined whether RIP reduces *S. aureus* adherence to human cells and dialysis catheters *in vitro* and observed that this peptide reduced adherence and biofilm formation not only on polyethylene catheters, but also on polyurethane and silicone catheters, with a predominant effect on silicone, to which *S. aureus* was more adherent. The authors concluded that RIP opens a new perspective in anti-staphylococcal prophylaxis, particularly in dialysis patients.

Conclusion

The present results support the hypothesis that RIP might be used for coating catheters in order to prevent colonization and consequent catheter-related infections. Thus, the prevention of biofilm formation by RIP may not only reduce infection rates, but also preserve the susceptibility of bacteria to antibiotics. Further studies regarding the prevention of CRBSI are necessary to clarify still unanswered questions, to help with decision making in view of existing controversies and to support the implementation of new technologies and their application in clinical practice, which will surely be reflected on the quality of care provided to patients with central venous catheters.

Acknowledgments

Fundação de Amparo a Pesquisa do Estado de São Paulo (FAPESP).

References

[1] O'Grady NP; Alexander, M; Dellinger, EP; Gerberding, JL; Heard, SO; Maki, DG; Masur, H; McCormick, RD; Mermel, LA; Pearson, ML; Raad, II; Randolph, A; Weinstein, RA. Centers for Disease Control and Prevention (CDC). Hospital Infection Control Practices Advisory Committee. CDC-*Guidelines for the Prevention of Intravascular Catheter-Related Infections*, 2002, MMWR 2002, 1(RR10), 1-26.

[2] Carrer, S; Bocchi, A; Bortolotti, M; Braga, N; Gilli, G; Candini, M; Tartari S. Effect of different sterile barrier precautions and central venous catheter dressing on the skin colonization around the insertion site. *Minerva Anestesiol*, 2005, 71, 197-206.

[3] Percival, SL; Kite, P; Eastwood, K; Murga, R; Carr, J; Arduino, MJ; Donlan, RM. Tetrasodium EDTA as a novel central venous catheter lock solution against biofilm. *Infect Control Hosp Epidemiol*, 2005, 26, 515-9.

[4] Bacuzzi, A; Cecchin, A; Del Bosco, A; Cantone, G; Cuffari, S. Recommendations and reports about central venous catheter-related infection. *Surg Infect (Larchmt)*, 2006, 7, S65-S7.

[5] Zamir, D; Polychuck, I; Leibovitz, I; Reitblat, T; Zamir, C; Schart, S. Nosocomial infections in internal medicine departaments. *Harefuah*, 2003, 142, 265-8.

[6] Warren, DK; Yokoe, DS; Climo, MW; Herwaldt, LA; Noskin, GA; Zuccotti, G; Tokars, JI; Perl, TM; Fraser, VJ. Preventing catheter-associated bloodstream infections: A survey of policies for insertion and care of central venous catheters from hospitals in the prevention epicenter program. *Infect Control Hosp Epidemiol*, 2006, 27, 8–13.

[7] Darouiche, RO. Prevention of vascular catheterrelated infections. *Neth J Med*, 1999, 55, 92-9.

[8] Beghetto, M; Victorino, J; Teixeira, L; Azevedo, M. Fatores de risco para infecção relacionada a cateter venoso central. *Rev Bras Ter Intensiva*, 2002, 14, 107-13.

[9] National Nosocomial Infections Surveillance System. National Nosocomial Infections Surveillance (NNIS) System report, data summary from January 1992 to June 2004, issued October 2004. *Am J Infect Control*, 2004, 32, 470-85.

[10] CDC. National Nosocomial Infections Surveillance (NNIS) System report, data summary from January 1990 - May 1999, issued June 1999. *Am J Infect Control*, 1999, 27, 520-32.

[11] Maki, DG. Infection caused by intravascular devices: Pathogenesis, strategies for prevention. Royal Society of Medicine Services Limited, London, England, 1991.

[12] Raad, II; Costerton, JW; Sabharwal, U; Sacilowski, M; Anaissie, E; Bodey, G. Ultrastructural analysis of indwelling vascular catheters: A quantitative relationship between luminal colonization and duration of placement. *J Infect Dis*, 168, 400-7, 1993.

[13] Kovalevich, DS; Faubion, WC; Bender, JM; Schaberg, DR; Wesley, JR. Association of parenteral nutrition catheter sepsis with urinary tract infections. *JPENJ Parenter Enteral Nutr*, 1986, 10, 639-41.

[14] CDC-Centers for Disease Control - *Nosocomial bacteremia associated with intravenous fluid therapy*. MMWR 20(suppl 9), S1-S2, 1971.

[15] Plouffe, JF; Brown, DG; Silva, J; Eck, T; Stricof, RL; Fekety, FR. Nosocomial outbreak of *Candida parapsilosis* fungemia related to intravenous infusions. *Arch Intern Med*, 1977. 137, 1686-99.

[16] Vaudaux, P; Pittet, D; Haeberli, A; Lerch, PG; Morgenthaler, JJ; Proctor, RA; Waldvogel, FA; Lew, DP. Fibronectin is more active than fibrin or fibrinogen in promoting *Staphylococcus aureus* adherence to inserted intravascular catheters. *J Infect Dis*, 1993, 167, 633-41.

[17] Cunha, MLRS, Caramori, JCT; Fioravante, AM; Batalha, JEN; Montelli, AC; Baretti, P. Significance of slime as Virulence Factor in Coagulase-Negative staphylococcus Peritonitis in CAPD. *Perit Dial Int*, 2004, 24, 191-3.

[18] Andes, D; Nett, J; Oschel, P; Albrecht, R; Marchillo, K; Pitula, A. 2004. Development and characterization of an in vivo central venous catheter *Candida albicans* biofilm model. *Infect. Immun*, 2004, 72, 6023-31.

[19] Collignon, PJ; Wilkinson, IJ; Gilbert, GL; Grayson, ML; Whitby, RM. Health care-associated *Staphylococcus aureus* bloodstream infections: a clinical quality indicator for all hospitals. *Med J Aust*, 2006, 184, 404-6.

[20] Lobo, RD; Levin, AS; Gomes, LM; Cursino, R; Park, M; Figueiredo, VB. Taniguchi, L; Polido, CG; Costa, SF. Impact of an educational program and policy changes on decreasing catheter-associated bloodstream infections in a medical intensive care unit in Brazil. *Am J Infect Control*, 2005, 33, 83-7.

[21] Yilmaz, G; Caylan, R; Aydin, K; Topbas, M; Koksal, I. Effect of education on the rate of and the understanding of risk factors for intravascular catheter-related infections. *Infect Control Hosp Epidemiol*, 2007, 28, 689-94.

[22] Pearson, ML. Guideline for prevention of intravascular-device- related infections. U.S. Department of Human Health and Human Services. Centers for Disease Control and Prevention. *Infect Control Hosp Epidemiol*, 1996, 17, 438-73.

[23] Elliott, TS; Moss, HA; Tebbs, SE; Wilson, IC; Bonser, RS; Graham, TR; Burke, LP; Faroqui, MH. Novel approach to investigate a source of microbial contamination of central venous catheters. *Eur J Clin Microbiol Infect Dis*, 1997, 16, 210–213.

[24] Drucker, DE; Greenfield, LJ; Ehrlich, F; Salzberg, AM. Aorto-iliac aneurysms following umbilical artery catheterization. *J Pediatr Surg*, 1986, 21, 725-30.

[25] Eiff, C; Jansen, B; Kohnen, W; Becker, K. Infections associated with medical devices: pathogenesis, management and prophylaxis. *Drugs*, 2005, 65, 179-214.

[26] Dezfulian, C; Lavelle, J; Nallamothu, BK; Kaufman, SR; Saint, S. Rates of infection for single-lumen versus multilumen central venous catheters: a meta-analysis. *Crit Care Med*, 2003, 31, 2385-90.

[27] Young, E; Commiskey, M; Wilson, S. Translating evidence into practice to prevent central venous catheter-associated bloodstream infections: A systems-based intervention. *Am J Infect Control*, 2006, 34, 503 – 6.

[28] Chaiyakunapruk, N; Veenstra, DL; Lipsky, BA; Saint, S. Chlorhexidine compared with povidone-iodine solution for vascular catheter-site care: a meta-analysis. *Ann Intern Med* 2002, 136, 792-801.

[29] Goetz, AM; Wagener, MM; Miller, JM; Muder, RR. Risk of infection due to central venous catheters: effect of site of placement and catheter type. *Infect Control Hosp Epidemiol*, 1998, 19, 842-5.

[30] Merrer, J; De Jonghe, B; Golliot, F; Lefrant, JY; Raffy, B; Barre, E; Rigaud, JP; Casciani, D; Misset, B; Bosquet, C; Outin, H; Brun-Buisson, C; Nitenberg, G; Complications of femoral and subclavian venous catheterization in critically ill patients: a randomized controlled trial. *JAMA*, 2001, 286, 700-7.

[31] Bijma, R; Girbes, AR; Kleijer, DJ; Zwaveling, JH. Preventing central venous catheter-related infection in a surgical intensive-care unit. *Infect Control Hosp Epidemiol*, 1999, 20, 618 -20.

[32] Mermel, LA. Prevention of intravascular catheter-related infections. *Ann Intern Med* 2000, 132, 391-402.

[33] Veenstra, DL; Saint, S; Saha, S; Lumley, T; Sullivan, SD. Efficacy of antiseptic-impregnated central venous catheters in preventing catheter-related bloodstream infection: a meta-analysis. *JAMA*, 1999, 281, 261-7.

[34] Maki, DG; Stolz, SM; Wheeler, S; Mermel, LA. Prevention of central venous catheter-related bloodstream infection by use of an antiseptic-impregnated catheter: a randomized, controlled trial. *Ann Intern Med*, 1997, 127, 257-66.

[35] Raad, II; Darouiche, R; Hachem, R; Mansouri, M; Bodey, GP. The broad-spectrum activity and efficacy of catheters coated with minocycline and rifampin. *J Infect Dis*, 1996, 173, 418-24.

[36] Bassetti, S; Hu, J; D'Agostino, RB Jr; Sherertz, RJ. Prolonged antimicrobial activity of a catheter containing chlorhexidine-silver sulfadiazine extends protection against catheter infections in vivo. *Antimicrob Agents Chemother*, 2001, 45, 1535-8.

[37] Oda, T; Hamasaki, J; Kanda, N; Mikami, K. Anaphylactic shock induced by an antiseptic-coated central venous catheter. *Anesthesiology*, 1997, 87, 1242-4.

[38] Veenstra, DL; Saint, S; Sullivan, SD. Cost-effectiveness of antiseptic-impregnated central venous catheters for the prevention of catheter-related bloodstream infection. *JAMA*, 1999, 282, 554-60.

[39] Raad, II; Buzaid, A; Ryne, J; et al. Minocycline and ethylenediaminetetraacetate for the prevention of recurrent vascular catheter infections. *Clin Infect Dis*, 1997, 25, 149-151 .

[40] Raad, II; Hachem, R; Sherertz, R: Minocycline-EDTA (M-EDTA) flush solution for the prevention of vascular catheter infection. In Program and Abstracts of the 34th Interscience *Conference on Antimicrobial Agents and Chemotherapy*, Orlando, Fla., 1994, Abstract J57, p 69.

[41] Randolph, AG; Cook, DJ; Gonzales, CA; Andrew, M. Benefit of heparin in central venous and pulmonary artery catheters: a meta-analysis of randomized controlled trials. *Chest* 1998, 113, 165-71.

[42] Schwartz, C; Henrickson, KJ; Roghmann, K; Powell, K. Prevention of bacteremia attributed to luminal colonization of tunneled central venous catheters with vancomycin-susceptible organisms. *J Clin Oncol*, 1990, 8, 591-7.

[43] Reardon, DM; Warner, B; Trowbridge, EA: EDTA; the traditional anticoagulant of haematology: With increased automation is it time for review? *Med Lab Sci*1991, 48, 72-5.

[44] Bleyer, A; Mason, L; Raad, I; Sherertz, R. A randomized, double-blind trial comparing minocycline/EDTA vs heparin as flush solutions for hemodialysis catheters. In: Program and abstracts of the Fourth Decennial Conference Program Committee; March 5-9, 2000, Atlanta, Ga. Abstract P-S1-31.

[45] Marconi, C; Cunha, MLRS; Lyra, JC; Bentlin, MR; Batalha, JEN; Sugizaki, MF; Rugolo, LMSS. Comparison between qualitative and semiquantitative catheter-tip cultures: laboratory diagnosis of catheter-related infection in newborns. *Braz. J. Microbiol*, 2008, 39, 262-7, 2008.

[46] Maki, DG; Weise, CE; Sarafin, HW. A semiquantitative culture method for identifying intravenous-catheter-related infection. *N. Engl. J. Med*, 1977, 296, 1305-09.

[47] Marconi, C; Cunha, MLRS; Lyra, JC; Bentlin, MR; Batalha, JEN; Sugizaki, MF; Corrente, JE; Rugolo, LMSS. Catheter tip culture utility in the diagnosis of neonatal infections. *J Pediatr* (*Rio J*), In Press, 2009.

[48] Bouza, E; Juan, RS; Muñoz, P; Pascau, J; Voss, A; Desco M. A European perspective on intravascular catheter-related infections: report on the microbiology workload, aetiology and antimicrobial susceptibility (ESGNI-005 Study). *Clin Microbiol Infect Dis*, 2004, 10, 838-42.

[49] Bruinson, C; Rauss, A; Legrand, P. Semiquantitative culture of catheter tips. *J Clin Microbiol*, 1987, 25, 1343-4.

[50] Capdevila, JA; Planes, AM; Palomar, M; Gasser, I; Almirante, D; Paissa, A; Crespo, E; Vazquez, JM Value of differential quantitative blood cultures in the diagnosis of catheter-related sepsis. *Eur J Clin Microbiol Infect Dis*, 1992, 11, 403-7.

[51] Blot, F; Nitenberg, G; Chachaty, E; et al. Diagnosis of catheter-related bacteremia: a prospective comparison of the time to positivity of hub-blood versus peripheral-blood cultures. *Lancet*, 1999, 354, 1071-7.

[52] Christensen, GD; Bisno, AL; Simpsom, WA; Beachey, EH. Adherence of slime producing strains of *Staphylococcus epidermidis* to smooth surfaces. *Infect. Immun*, 1982, 37, 318-26.

[53] Freeman, DJ; Falkner, FR; KEANE, CT. New method for detecting slime production by coagulase-negative staphylococci. *J Clin Pathol*, 1989, 42, 872-4.

[54] Garvis, S; Mei, JM; Ruiz-Albert, J; Holden, DW. *Staphylococcus aureus svrA*: a gene required for virulence and expression of the *agr* locus. *Microbiology*, 2002, 148, 3235–43.

[55] Balaban, N; Collins, LV; Cullor, JS; Hume, EB; Medina-Acosta, E; Motta, OV; O'Callaghan, R; Rossitto, PV; Shirtliff, ME; Silveira, LS; Tarkowski, A; Torres, JV. 2000. Prevention of diseases caused by *Staphylococcus aureus* using the peptide RIP. *Peptides*, 2000, 21, 1301-11.

[56] Balaban, N; Gov Y; Bitler A; Boelaert JR. Prevention of *Staphylococcus aureus* biofilm on dialysis catheters and adherence to human cells. *Kidney Int*. 2003, 63, 340-5.

[57] Balaban, N; Giacometti, A; Cirioni, O; Gov, Y; Ghiselli, R; Mocchegiani, F; Viticchi, C; Del Prete, MS; Saba, V; Scalise, G; Dell'Acqua, G. Use of the quorum-sensing inhibitor RNAIII-inhibiting peptide to prevent biofilm formation in vivo by drug-resistant *Staphylococcus epidermidis*. *J Infect Dis*, 2003, 187, 625-630.

In: Cross Infections: Types, Causes and Prevention
Editors: Jin Dong and Xun Liang

ISBN: 978-1-60741-467-4
© 2009 Nova Science Publishers, Inc.

Chapter IV

Surveillance for Healthcare-Associated Infections in Pediatric Cancer Patients: An Important Prerequisite of Ongoing Prevention and Quality Control

Arne Simon*
Children's Hospital Medical Center University of Bonn, Germany

Introduction

Pediatric cancer patients face an increased risk of potentially life-threatening infectious complications [1-4] due to their underlying malignancy and to the adverse effects of intensive anticancer treatment [5-7]. The most important risk factor for infection in these patients is the duration of severe neutropenia [8, 9], which has been defined as an absolute neutrophil count $< 0.5 \times 10^9/L$ or as a decreasing leukocyte count $< 1.0 \times 10^9/L$ without a differential count available.

The majority of infections observed during intensive treatment in pediatric cancer patients are bloodstream infections (BSIs) [10]. Many of these potentially life threatening events are associated with the use of long term central venous access devices (CVAD) [11-14].

In this context, the term 'healthcare-associated infection' (HAI) refers to infectious complications in a specific group of patients, who suffer from chronic underlying disease (malignancy) and depend on medical support for a prolonged time period (months or even years). These patients are often immunocompromised and in close contact with in- and outpatient professional medical care services. The term HAI is more appropriate to describe the real life situation of pediatric cancer patients than the traditional term of 'nosocomial infection', which refers only to those events, which have been acquired in the hospital.

*Corresponding Author: Priv. Doz. Dr. med. Arne Simon Children's Hospital Medical Center University of Bonn Adenauerallee 119, 53113 Bonn, Germany Tel +49-22828733254 Fax +49-22828733301 Email asimon@ukb.uni-bonn.de

Surveillance is defined as ongoing, systematic collection, analysis, interpretation, and dissemination [15] of data regarding HAIs for the description of endemic infection rates and incidence densities and for the promotion of targeted preventive measures to reduce HAI related morbidity, mortality and resource utilization´[16, 17]. Although much can be learned from outbreak investigations [18-21] how gaps in barrier precautions and failures in preventive efforts can be overcome, they do not give us valid information about the endemic HAI rate. It is a consensus between experts, that outbreaks represent only the minor proportion of all NI [22-25].

Healthcare-associated infections (HAIs) in pediatric cancer patients have been investigated only in a few single-center studies [12, 26-28]. One additional European study included two pediatric oncology units [29] in a 6-month prospective survey using periodic chart review during hospitalization, but did not use adjusted definitions for immunocompromised pediatric patients [30]. The exact proportion of HAIs in these high-risk patients is unknown; two single-center prospective studies in pediatric hematology-oncology patients, excluding allogenic bone marrow transplantations, found an incidence of 20% [26] [incidence density (ID) 10.8/1,000 inpatient days] and 24% [27] (ID 17.7/1,000 inpatient days), respectively.

One recent single-center study found an ID of 38.9 HAIs per 1,000 inpatient days in a pediatric stem-cell and bone-marrow transplantation unit [28], but the corresponding protocol referred only to treatment periods with neutropenia [31].

In 1998, our group developed a module for the prospective unit-based surveillance of HAI in pediatric cancer patients: Onkopaed NKI. The results of a prospective single-center 10-month pilot study confirmed the feasibility of this module as well as the high risk of HAI and CVAD-associated BSIs in pediatric cancer patients [26].

In the meantime, the Onkopaed NKI module has been used for prospective intervention studies on CVAD-associated infections [32], the restricted use of glycopeptides as a component of empirical antimicrobial therapy [33], antifungal prophylaxis with itraconazole [34], and the prevention of CVAD-associated Gram-positive infections (Coagulase-negative staphylococci) with a taurolidine containing lock solution [35]. Recently, our group published the results of the first prospective multicenter surveillance study of HAI in pediatric cancer patients using standardized CDC methods and adjusted consensus definitions for this special patient population, performed in 7 pediatric oncology centers from Germany and Switzerland [36].

Herein, we would like to comment on what we have learned during 10 years of prospective surveillance of HAIs in pediatric cancer patients in order to let other pediatric oncologists and infectious disease specialists take part in and benefit from our experiences.

What is the Primary Purpose of Prospective Surveillance?

The primary purpose of prospective surveillance of HAIs is to provide the pediatric oncology treatment team with robust data on the distribution and the incidence density of selected adverse infectious complications, which are of outstanding clinical relevance and may be, at least in part, be preventable by specific interventions. The interim results of any surveillance project should timely be fed back to the decision makers in primary medical care [15]. According to the local structures and responsibilities, the stakeholders (physicians, health care workers, administrative personnel, microbiologists and infection control personnel, hospital epidemiologists) should actively use these data to scrutinize the effectiveness of the current practice of infection prevention and control regularly [24, 37]. During prospective continuous surveillance, these data can be used to investigate the effects of specific interventions [38-41].

Use Adapted Definitions

Surveillance of HAIs in pediatric cancer patients should rely on a set of adapted definitions [30], which take the diagnostic obstacles in immunocompromised patients into account and broaden the scope of the documented events for example to certain invasive fungal infections, which are extremely rare in other pediatric patient populations. The complete set of definitions, developed for our pilot study [26] and utilized in our multicentre surveillance protocol [36] may be achieved from the author of this chapter by email request.

Surveillance Should not be Restricted to Periods of Neutropenia

Although associated with a severe clinical course, a significant proportion of all pediatric cancer patients with HAI do not have neutropenia at the time of diagnosis [36]. This is in agreement with results from other groups who found severe CVAD-related infections in pediatric cancer patients in the absence of neutropenia [42, 43]. As a consequence, surveillance should not be limited to the period of neutropenia, and for the calculation of IDs days of neutropenia should not be used as the (sole) denominator. In addition, it is important to include late infections after stem cell transplantation (> 40 days after Tx), in particular invasive aspergillosis in patients without neutropenia, but with severe graft versus host disease [44, 45]

Surveillance Should Focus on Microbiologically Confirmed Infections

Of 727 events, 263 (36%; 181 patients) were HAIs and 464 (64%; 230 patients) were fevers of unknown origin (FUO) [36]. The surveillance of HAIs in pediatric oncology patients, where FUO accounts for at least 60% of all episodes of febrile neutropenia [27, 28], can only yield reliable results, if each individual episode of fever is subject to a meticulous analysis, searching for a HAI, according to the definitions of the surveillance protocol [46]. On the other hand, it remains an unresolved issue, how FUO can be prevented in patients treated with intensive chemotherapy.

In addition, the detailed documentation of all FUO events drains resources, which could be better invested in preventive activities as the education of patients and their parents in the most important modes of transmission and the prevention of hospital acquired infections by simple basic hygiene (hand disinfection, adequate use of glows and masks, prevention of infections related to food items [47], and basic preventive rules for outpatient treatment periods at home, e.g. during social activities or after pet contacts [48]. Profound information of the patients and their families may also increase the compliance considering the use of specific medication for antibacterial and antifungal prophylaxis [49].

Taken together, in times of very restricted time budgets and limited availability of infection control personnel, surveillance should focus on a thoroughly selected set of events, which are epidemiologically and economically relevant in clinical practice and represent microbiologically confirmed infections.

Prospective Surveillance and Interventions to Reduce CVAD-Associated Infections

Since CVAD-associated BSI represent a major proportion of all HAI in pediatric cancer patients [11, 57], all practical opportunities to prevent these adverse events should be followed. The aim of 'zero tolerance' for intravenous catheter-related infections has been defined for intensive care patients with short term central venous catheters [58], and some advocates have recently set this new target for cancer patients, too [59].

Pediatric oncology units should follow a written policy for the prevention of CVAD-related infections which translates the available evidence considering all critical control points of catheter insertion and catheter care into clinical practice [60-62]. These efforts should be an integral part of a 'population-based' infection control intervention program, focusing not only on the prevention of BSIs, but also on good hand hygiene practice [63], prevention of nosocomial pneumonia [64], gastrointestinal infections [18, 65], and surgical site infections [66], as well as environmental cleaning and disinfection [67, 68].

It remains important to differentiate three types of BSI in patients with a CVAD:

- Confirmed CVAD-related infection (the CVAD is the confirmed source of the infection);
- CVAD-associated infection (fever or other clinical signs of infection with a positive blood culture drawn from the CVAD in a patient without another apparent focus of infection);
- Secondary BSI in a patient with a CVAD (another source of bacteremia has been confirmed by physical examination, microbiological methods, sonography, X-ray, computer tomography or magnetic resonance imaging).

Important examples for secondary bacteremias are sepsis due to viridans streptococci in patients with neutropenia and severe chemotherapy-induced mucositis [69] or *Gram*-negative bacteremias with pathogens derived from the patient's gut in patients with leukemia and anorectal ulcerations [70].

Most surveillance tools document CVAD-associated infections and normalize the results to 1000 utilization days (incidence density) [71, 72]. While interpreting the results, one has to consider, which utilization days have been used as denominator: only inpatient utilization days [26, 36] or all utilization days from the date of implantation to the date of removal of the CVAD [73].

One observation of our pilot study was a much higher incidence density of CVAD-associated infections during inpatient treatment periods (7.4 vs. 0.3 / 1000 utilization days; relative risk 21; $p < 0.001$). There is much more manipulation of the CVAD and the different components of the i.v. system [32] during inpatient treatment periods [74]. Thus, it seems reasonable to focus the prospective surveillance on inpatient utilization days. CVAD utilization days as well as other basic data (inpatient days, number of admissions to the unit, acute transplantation days) may easily be documented every midnight (only those patients, who stay in the unit over night are counted as inpatients).

One important consideration in this context is the number of utilization days to be expected for a certain CVAD type in a defined time period of surveillance. Incidence densities display pronounced variations as long as the number of utilization days is lower than at least 1000 per device. Therefore, it may take many months or even a year to derive valid and informative data on the unit epidemiology of device-associated infections related to a device, which is only rarely used in the patients of this particular unit. This advisement prompted us to renounce the surveillance of urinary tract infections related to urinary tract catheters or of central nervous system infections related to an external CNS drainage, since the utilization rates for both devices are to low in our patient population.

If an outbreak is suspected from the interpretation of the CVAD-associated infection data, more detailed diagnostic efforts, which are beyond the scope of this article, should be implemented to confirm the CVAD as the source of the infection [11, 75].

Continuously performed prospective surveillance of CVAD-associated BSIs adds the opportunity to investigate the benefit of specific interventions. Two examples for such an intervention are the intermittent use of urokinase and antimicrobial locks of the internal catheter lumen with taurolidine.

Fibrin deposition at the intraluminal surface of the indwelling part of the central venous catheter (CVC) surface increases the risk of CVC-related coagulase-negative staphylococci (CoNS) infection. Therefore, repetitive enzymatic dissolution of fibrin by urokinase might reduce the risk of CVC-related infection [76, 77]. Two randomized studies confirmed a benefit of urokinase administration or in terms of prevention considering *Gram*-positive catheter-associated infections. The different regimens were urokinase 5,000 U/mL in a volume sufficient to fill the entire device every 2 weeks [78] and 25,000 U in 5 mL three times weekly [79]. In one of both studies, which investigated tunneled external catheters as well as infusion ports, the protective effect did demonstrate statistical significance only in external catheters [78].

In the study of van Rooden et al., other secondary complications, including CVC-related thrombosis, were observed less frequently in the urokinase group compared with the placebo group (1.3% v 9.0%, respectively; RR = 0.14; 95% CI, 0.02 to 0.82).

Our group recently published a single center prospective 48-months cohort study [35] in patients receiving anticancer chemotherapy from April 2003 to March 2005 (group 1, heparin lock with 200 IU/ml sterile normal saline 0.9%; Canusal® Wockhardt UK Ltd, Wrexham, Wales) were compared to all patients from April 2005 to March 2007 (group 2; taurolidine 1.35%/Sodium Citrate 4%; TauroLock™,Tauropharm, Waldbüttelbrunn, Germany). Taurolidin/Citrate (TauroLock™) is a non-toxic lock solution with broad spectrum antimicrobial activity and citrate as anticoagulant, which has been shown to prevent catheter-related infections in dialysis patients [80, 81] and in patients on long term home parenteral nutrition [82]. In group 1 (heparin), 90 patients had 98 CVAD in use during the surveillance period. 14 of 30 (47%) BSI were 'primary Gram positive BSI due to Coagulase-negative staphylococci (CoNS) (n = 4) or or Methicillin-resistent *Staphylococcus epidermidis* (MRSE) (n = 10)' [incidence density (ID); 2.30 per 1000 inpatient CVAD-utilization days].

In group 2 (TauroLock™), 89 patients had 95 CVAD in use during the surveillance period. 3 of 25 (12%) BSI were caused by CoNS. (ID, 0.45). The difference in the ID between the two groups was statistically significant (P = 0.004). In our unit the routine use of Taurolidine lock solution prevented 6 CVAD-related *Gram*-positive infections (due to CoNS or MRSE) per year.

In a subsequent matched-pairs study, which has been submitted for publication, the additional cost of one BSI in our pediatric oncology unit was very conservatively calculated to be 4.440 Euro (IQR 3.145 – 5.920 Euro); in terms of prevention, the routine use of Taurolidine lock solution resulted in cost savings of € 26,000 (IQR € 18,800–35,400) per year, and the prevention of only two BSIs per year would balance the acquisition cost of TauroLock™.

Respiratory Tract Infections

In the majority of patients in our multicentre study with radiologically confirmed pneumonia, no causative agent could be identified. This is the consequence of restricted opportunities of invasive diagnostic methods as bronchoalveolar lavage or lung biopsy in patients outside the stem cell transplant setting [28, 50]. Nasopharyngel aspirate represents an easy obtainable diagnostic material for the diagnosis of viral respiratory tract infections. Most pediatric oncology units work in close cooperation with virology laboratories and should use the state of the art diagnostic tools as (rt)PCR [51, 52] to identify viral pathogens from respiratory secretions of children with symptoms of respiratory tract infection [53].

Although the spectrum of therapeutic interventions is still rather limited [54], these pathogens can easily be transmitted from patient to patient and thus require barrier precautions and isolation to prevent nosocomial outbreaks [55, 56].

Gastrointestinal Infections

Based on our experience with a Norovirus outbreak in pediatric oncology patients [18] and our recent investigation of Rotavirus infections in a matched pairs analysis [65], the surveillance of gastrointestinal HAI in pediatric cancer patients should at least cover infections due to Norovirus, Rotavirus, and *Clostridium difficile*-associated diseases (CDAD), The latter is, however, difficult to define in this population, since diarrhea, abdominal pain and even colitis may be an adverse effect of chemotherapy or local radiation (mucositis) [83]. Our results confirmed the observation of Dettenkofer et al. [31] that a remarkable proportion (30-70%) of all symptomatic patients with CDAD do not suffer from neutropenia at the time of diagnosis. The empirical antimicrobial regimen of fever and neutropenia does not cover *C. difficile* and fosters the production of *C. difficile* toxins [84]. Discontinuation of the offending antibiotic as a general treatment principle in patients with CDAD [85] is not feasible in patients with neutropenia. Recently, hypervirulent nosocomially transmitted *C. difficile* isolates have been described in several countries, causing increased morbidity, length of hospital stay, and mortality in adult patients [86]. Considering the significant morbidity of affected patients, the possibility of outbreaks, and the emerging threat of hypervirulent isolates, it seems mandatory to implement continuous prospective surveillance of CDAD in pediatric cancer patients [87]. In our multicentre study, *Clostridium difficile* associated disease (CDAD) was defined as symptoms of an abdominal infection starting at least 48 hours after hospital admission, and with a positive *C. difficile*-toxin cell culture assay from at least one stool specimen, leading to initiation of antimicrobial treatment directed against *C. difficile* for at least 5 days [36]. In total, 24 cases of CDAD were reported. In 3 patients, surgical interventions were necessary during the clinical course of the acute intra-abdominal infection. In one center, 9 out of 13 cases were reported from June, 2001 to January, 2001, for an incidence density of 3.79 (9 events in 2,376 inpatient days). After the local preventive measures were reorganized [88], the ID decreased to 0.44 (4 cases in 9,077 days).

Invasive Fungal Infections

Still a matter of great concern is the high mortality [89] in patients with invasive aspergillosis [44], in particular in those patients with disseminated disease or with central nervous system involvement.

The recognition of the role of external reservoirs [90] and acute exposure to fungal spores [91] as well as the broadening scope of the agents available for antifungal prophylaxis [34, 92-94] may contribute to a higher success rate in the prevention of these often fatal infection in high risk pediatric cancer patients.

Nonetheless, it is necessary to supply the treatment team regularly with prospectively collected data on the local unit epidemiology in order to identify any possible outbreak (2 ore more patients, temporally related) as soon as possible and to evaluate the efficacy of the local regimen of antifungal prophylaxis [34].

Multiresistant Isolates

The proportion of resistant BSI-isolates in our multicentre study [36] was surprisingly low, considering the increasing proportion of resistant isolates in studies from other countries [29]. Wisplinghof et al. [95] determined antimicrobial susceptibilities of nosocomial BSI isolates in pediatric patients in the US SCOPE project. As in our study, Gram-positive pathogens accounted for most (65%) of the cases, Gram-negative pathogens for 24% and fungi for 11%. We identified only a single case of candidemia. In Wisplinghof's study, the proportion of MRSA increased from 10% in 1995 to 29% in 2001 [95]. Vancomycin-resistance was seen in 11% of *E. faecium* isolates (VRE). In our study, no BSI was caused by MRSA, but 2 of 5 *E. faecium* BSI were caused by VRE.

In the study of Raymond et al. [29], the prevalence of antimicrobial resistance depended on the type of unit. Up to 26% of *S. aureus* and 89% of CoNS were methicillin-resistant (MRSA, MRSE), and 38% of *K. pneumoniae* expressed an extended-spectrum beta-lactamase (ESBL) [96]. One positive side effect of prospective surveillance is the regular provision of contemporary data on antimicrobial susceptibility patterns of important pathogens related to HAIs [97, 98].

Documentation of Objective Outcome Parameters

In particular from the perspective of resource consumption related to HAIs, the case report forms of the surveillance tool should ask for objective outcome parameters:

- Surgical removal of a CVAD related to the infection;
- Necessity of other surgical interventions (e.g. in patients with infections associated with orthopedic implants [99], severe CDAD [100] or with invasive aspergillosis [101];
- The use of expensive antibiotics and antimycotics;
- The duration of inpatient ad outpatient treatment related to the infection;
- The duration of intensive care treatment and of mechanical ventilation;
- The attributable mortality (after consensus discussion with the attending pediatric oncologists).

Information of All Contributors and Stakeholders

The pediatric oncology treatment team is very interested and willing to spent time and personnel efforts in any improvement of hygiene precautions which may lead to a reduction of HAI [102]. In particular pediatric oncology nurses are confronted with the adverse consequences of HAIs 'at the bedside' of the patients, they care for [103, 104].

In contrast, hospital pharmacists and financial controlling administrators may prefer to analyze the problem from the perspective of increased resource utilization and cost (use of expensive antibiotics and antifungals, prolonged length of stay, need for intensive care ore surgical interventions) [105-107].

Prospective surveillance depends on financial and personnel resources and thus, the concept of the surveillance protocol and the cost of surveillance activities should be discussed upfront with all stakeholders and decision makers from the different occupational groups participating in clinical care for pediatric cancer patients.

Conclusion

Today, HAIs are considered to be important adverse outcomes in terms of increased morbidity and mortality, postponed chemotherapy treatment cycles, as well as prolonged duration of hospital stay and additional costs from the perspective of the caregiver. All efforts to prevent HAI and to contain the nosocomial spread of pathogens are critical aspects of patient's safety in the hospital environment [108]. Thus, the prospective surveillance of HAI should be recognized as a fundamental component of quality assurance and control in the treatment of immunocompromised pediatric cancer patients. Pediatric oncologists, pediatric infectious disease specialists, and infection control personnel should combine their efforts and work together improving the quality of supportive care and eliminating the preventable proportion of HAIs in pediatric oncology departments [109, 110].

References

[1] Haupt, R; Romanengo, M; Fears, T; Viscoli, C; Castagnola, E. Incidence of septicaemias and invasive mycoses in children undergoing treatment for solid tumours: a 12-year experience at a single Italian institution. *Eur J Cancer,* 2001, 37(18), 2413-9.

[2] Castagnola, E; Cesaro, S; Giacchino, M; Livadiotti, S; Tucci, F; Zanazzo, G; et al. Fungal infections in children with cancer: a prospective, multicenter surveillance study. *Pediatr Infect Dis J*, 2006, 25(7), 634-9.

[3] Castagnola, E; Conte, M; Parodi, S; Papio, F; Caviglia, I; Haupt, R. Incidence of bacteremias and invasive mycoses in children with high risk neuroblastoma. *Pediatr Blood Cancer*, 2007, 49(5), 672-7.

[4] Castagnola, E; Fratino, G; Valera, M; Giacchino, M; Haupt, R; Molinari, AC. Correlation between "malfunctioning events" and catheter-related infections in pediatric cancer patients bearing tunneled indwelling central venous catheter: results of a prospective observational study. *Support Care Cancer*, 2005.

[5] Gaur, AH; Flynn, PM; Shenep, JL. Optimum management of pediatric patients with fever and neutropenia. *Indian J Pediatr*, 2004, 71(9), 825-35.

[6] Neville, K; Renbarger, J; Dreyer, Z. Pneumonia in the immunocompromised pediatric cancer patient. *Semin Respir Infect*, 2002, 17(1), 21-32.

[7] Benjamin, DK; Jr.; Miller, WC; Bayliff, S; Martel, L; Alexander, KA; Martin, PL. Infections diagnosed in the first year after pediatric stem cell transplantation. *Pediatr Infect Dis J*, 2002, 21(3), 227-34.

[8] Lehrnbecher, T; Foster, C; Vazquez, N; Mackall, CL; Chanock, SJ. Therapy-induced alterations in host defense in children receiving therapy for cancer. *J Pediatr Hematol Oncol*, 1997, 19(5), 399-417.

[9] Bodey, G; Buckley, M; Sathe, Y; Freireich, EJ. Quantitative relationships between circulating leukocytes and infection in patients with acute leukemia. *Ann Intern Med*, 1966, 64, 328-40.

[10] Adler, A; Yaniv, I; Steinberg, R; Solter, E; Samra, Z; Stein, J; et al. Infectious complications of implantable ports and Hickman catheters in paediatric haematology-oncology patients. *J Hosp Infect*, 2006, 62(3), 358-65.

[11] Simon, A; Bode, U; Beutel, K. Diagnosis and treatment of catheter-related infections in paediatric oncology: an update. *Clin Microbiol Infect*, 2006, 12(7), 606-20.

[12] Paulus, SC; van Saene, HK; Hemsworth, S; Hughes, J; Ng, A; Pizer, BL. A prospective study of septicaemia on a paediatric oncology unit: a three-year experience at The Royal Liverpool Children's Hospital, Alder Hey, UK. *Eur J Cancer*, 2005, 41(14), 2132-40.

[13] Castagnola, E; Molinari, AC; Giacchino, M; Chiapello, N; Moroni, C; Caviglia, I; et al. Incidence of catheter-related infections within 30 days from insertion of Hickman-Broviac catheters. *Pediatr Blood Cancer*, 2007, 48(1), 35-8.

[14] Viscoli, C; Castagnola, E; Giacchino, M; Cesaro, S; Properzi, E; Tucci, F; et al. Bloodstream infections in children with cancer: a multicentre surveillance study of the Italian Association of Paediatric Haematology and Oncology. Supportive Therapy Group-Infectious Diseases Section. *Eur J Cancer,* 1999, 35(5), 770-4.

[15] Gaynes, R; Richards, C; Edwards, J; Emori, TG; Horan, T; Alonso-Echanove, J; et al. Feeding back surveillance data to prevent hospital-acquired infections. *Emerg Infect Dis*, 2001, 7(2), 295-8.
[16] Centers for Disease Control and Prevention. Updated guidelines for evaluating public health surveillance systems: recommendations from the guidelines working group. *Morbidity and Mortality Weekly Report*, 2001, 50(RR-13), 1-51.
[17] Tokars, JI; Richards, C; Andrus, M; Klevens, M; Curtis, A; Horan, T; et al. The changing face of surveillance for health care-associated infections. *Clin Infect Dis*, 2004, 39(9), 1347-52.
[18] Simon, A; Schildgen, O; Maria Eis-Hubinger, A; Hasan, C; Bode, U; Buderus, S; et al. Norovirus outbreak in a pediatric oncology unit. *Scand J Gastroenterol*, 2006, 41(6), 693-9.
[19] Buttery, JP; Alabaster, SJ; Heine, RG; Scott, SM; Crutchfield, RA; Bigham, A; et al. Multiresistant Pseudomonas aeruginosa outbreak in a pediatric oncology ward related to bath toys. *Pediatr Infect Dis J*, 1998, 17(6), 509-13.
[20] Kline, S; Cameron, S; Streifel, A; Yakrus, MA; Kairis, F; Peacock, K; et al. An outbreak of bacteremias associated with Mycobacterium mucogenicum in a hospital water supply. Infect *Control Hosp Epidemiol*, 2004, 25(12), 1042-9.
[21] Kappstein, I; Grundmann, H; Hauer, T; Niemeyer, C. Aerators as a reservoir of Acinetobacter junii: an outbreak of bacteraemia in paediatric oncology patients. *J Hosp Infect*, 2000, 44(1), 27-30.
[22] Gastmeier, P; Stamm-Balderjahn, S; Hansen, S; Nietzschke-Tiemann, F; Zuschneid, I; Groneberg, K; et al. [Use of information on nosocomial outbreaks for infection control]. *Bundesgesundheitsblatt Gesundheitsforschung Gesundheitsschutz*, 2004, 47(4), 334-8.
[23] Kommission für Krankenhaushygiene und Infektionsprävention. Ausbruchsmanagement und strukturiertes Vorgehen bei gehäuftem Auftreten nosokomialer Infektionen. Empfehlung der Kommission für Krankenhaushygiene und Infektionsprävention am Robert Koch-Institut. *Bundesgesundheitsblatt - Gesundheitsforschung - Gesundheitsschutz*, 2002, 45(2), 180-6.
[24] Gastmeier, P; Sohr, D; Just, HM; Nassauer, A; Daschner, F; Ruden, H. How to survey nosocomial infections. *Infect Control Hosp Epidemiol*, 2000, 21(6), 366-70.
[25] Gastmeier, P; Vonberg, RP. Outbreaks of nosocomial infections: lessons learned and perspectives. *Curr Opin Infect Dis*, 2008, 21(4), 357-61.
[26] Simon, A; Fleischhack, G; Hasan, C; Bode, U; Engelhart, S; Kramer, MH. Surveillance for nosocomial and central line-related infections among pediatric hematology-oncology patients. *Infect Control Hosp Epidemiol*, 2000, 21(9), 592-6.
[27] Urrea, M; Rives, S; Cruz, O; Navarro, A; Garcia, JJ; Estella, J. Nosocomial infections among pediatric hematology/oncology patients: results of a prospective incidence study. *Am J Infect Control*, 2004, 32(4), 205-8.
[28] Laws, HJ; Kobbe, G; Dilloo, D; Dettenkofer, M; Meisel, R; Geisel, R; et al. Surveillance of nosocomial infections in paediatric recipients of bone marrow or peripheral blood stem cell transplantation during neutropenia, compared with adult recipients. *J Hosp Infect,* 2005.
[29] Raymond, J; Aujard, Y. Nosocomial infections in pediatric patients: a European, multicenter prospective study. European Study Group. *Infect Control Hosp Epidemiol*, 2000, 21(4), 260-3.

[30] Carlisle, PS; Gucalp, R; Wiernik, PH. Nosocomial infections in neutropenic cancer patients. *Infect Control Hosp Epidemiol*, 1993, 14(6), 320-4.

[31] Dettenkofer, M; Ebner, W; Bertz, H; Babikir, R; Finke, J; Frank, U; et al. Surveillance of nosocomial infections in adult recipients of allogeneic and autologous bone marrow and peripheral blood stem-cell transplantation. *Bone Marrow Transplant*, 2003, 31(9), 795-801.

[32] Simon, A; Fleischhack, G; Wiszniewsky, G; Hasan, C; Bode, U; Kramer, MH. Influence of Prolonged Use of Intravenous Administration Sets in Paediatric Cancer Patients on CVAD-related Bloodstream Infection Rates and Hospital Resources. *Infection*, 2006, 34(5), 258-63.

[33] Simon, A; Groger, N; Wilkesmann, A; Hasan, C; Wiszniewsky, G; Engelhart, S; et al. Restricted use of glycopeptides in paediatric cancer patients with fever and neutropenia. *Int J Antimicrob Agents,* 2006, 28(5), 417-22.

[34] Simon, A; Besuden, M; Vezmar, S; Hasan, C; Lampe, D; Kreutzberg, S; et al. Itraconazole prophylaxis in pediatric cancer patients receiving conventional chemotherapy or autologous stem cell transplants. *Support Care Cancer*, 2006, Aug 30 (Epub ahead of Print).

[35] Simon, A; Ammann, RA; Wiszniewsky, G; Bode, U; Fleischhack, G; Besuden, MM. Taurolidine-citrate lock solution (TauroLock™) significantly reduces CVAD-associated Gram positive infections in paediatric cancer patients. *BMC Infectious Diseases*, 2008, 8, 102 (29Jul2008)

[36] Simon, A; Ammann, RA; Bode, U; Fleischhack, G; Wenchel, HM; Schwamborn, D; et al. Nosocomial infections in pediatric cancer patients: results of a prospective surveillance study from 7 University hospitals in Germany and Switzerland. *BMC Infect Dis*, 2008, E-Pub May 23, 2008(8), 70.

[37] Gastmeier, P. Nosocomial infection surveillance and control policies. *Curr Opin Infect Dis*, 2004, 17(4), 295-301.

[38] Gaynes, RP. Surveillance of nosocomial infections: a fundamental ingredient for quality. *Infect Control Hosp Epidemiol*, 1997, 18(7), 475-8.

[39] Gastmeier, P; Sohr, D; Geffers, C; Nassauer, A; Daschner, F; Ruden, H. Are nosocomial infection rates in intensive care units useful benchmark parameters? *Infection*, 2000, 28(6), 346-50.

[40] Weinstein, RA; Siegel, JD; Brennan, PJ. Infection-control report cards--securing patient safety. *N Engl J Med*, 2005, 353(3), 225-7.

[41] Wong, ES; Rupp, ME; Mermel, L; Perl, TM; Bradley, S; Ramsey, KM; et al. Public disclosure of healthcare-associated infections: the role of the Society for Healthcare Epidemiology of America. *Infect Control Hosp Epidemiol*, 2005, 26(2), 210-2.

[42] Aledo, A; Heller, G; Ren, L; Gardner, S; Dunkel, I; McKay, SW; et al. Septicemia and septic shock in pediatric patients: 140 consecutive cases on a pediatric hematology-oncology service. *J Pediatr Hematol Oncol*, 1998, 20(3), 215-21.

[43] Gorelick, MH; Owen, WC; Seibel, NL; Reaman, GH. Lack of association between neutropenia and the incidence of bacteremia associated with indwelling central venous catheters in febrile pediatric cancer patients. *Pediatr Infect Dis J*, 1991, 10(7), 506-10.

[44] Groll, AH; Kurz, M; Schneider, W; Witt, V; Schmidt, H; Schneider, M; et al. Five-year-survey of invasive aspergillosis in a paediatric cancer centre. *Epidemiology, management and long-term survival. Mycoses*, 1999, 42(7-8), 431-42.

[45] Upton, A; Kirby, KA; Carpenter, P; Boeckh, M; Marr, KA. Invasive aspergillosis following hematopoietic cell transplantation: outcomes and prognostic factors associated with mortality. *Clin Infect Dis*, 2007, 44(4), 531-40.

[46] Simon, A; Bode, U; Fleischhack, G; Kramer, M. Surveillance of nosocomial infections in pediatric cancer patients. *Am J Infect Control*, 2005, 33(10), 611.

[47] Moody, K; Charlson, ME; Finlay, J. The neutropenic diet: what's the evidence? *J Pediatr Hematol Oncol*, 2002, 24(9), 717-21.

[48] Hemsworth, S; Pizer, B. Pet ownership in immunocompromised children--a review of the literature and survey of existing guidelines. *Eur J Oncol Nurs*, 2006, 10(2), 117-27.

[49] Lehrnbecher, T; Laws, HJ; Boehm, A; Dworzak, M; Janssen, G; Simon, A; et al. Compliance with anti-infective preventive measures: A multicentre survey among paediatric oncology patients. *Eur J Cancer*, 2008, 44(13), 1861-5.

[50] Zar, HJ; Cotton, MF. Nosocomial pneumonia in pediatric patients: practical problems and rational solutions. *Paediatr Drugs*, 2002, 4(2), 73-83.

[51] Simon, A; Volz, S; Fleischhack, G; Tillman, R; Muller, A; Bode, U; et al. Human coronavirus OC43 pneumonia in a pediatric cancer patient with down syndrome and acute lymphoblastic leukemia. *J Pediatr Hematol Oncol*, 2007, 29(6), 432-4.

[52] Watzinger, F; Suda, M; Preuner, S; Baumgartinger, R; Ebner, K; Baskova, L, et al. Real-time quantitative PCR assays for detection and monitoring of pathogenic human viruses in immunosuppressed pediatric patients. *J Clin Microbiol*, 2004, 42(11), 5189-98.

[53] Simon, A; Schildgen, O; Schuster, F. Viral infections in children with cancer. *Arch Dis Child*, 2008.

[54] Simon, A; Schildgen, O; Panning, M; Bode, U; Eis-Hubinger, A. RSV-infection in patients with cancer – still more questions than answers. *Clin Infect Dis*, 2008, 46(15 June), 1933-4.

[55] Simon, A; Khurana, K; Wilkesmann, A; Muller, A; Engelhart, S; Exner, M; et al. Nosocomial respiratory syncytial virus infection: Impact of prospective surveillance and targeted infection control. *Int J Hyg Environ Health*, 2006, 209(4), 317-24.

[56] Simon, A; Muller, A; Khurana, K; Engelhart, S; Exner, M; Schildgen, O; et al. Nosocomial infection: A risk factor for a complicated course in children with respiratory syncytial virus infection - Results from a prospective multicenter German surveillance study. Int *J Hyg Environ Health*, 2008, 211(3-4), 241-50.

[57] van Rooden, CJ; Schippers, EF; Barge, RM; Rosendaal, FR; Guiot, HF; van der Meer FJ; et al. Infectious complications of central venous catheters increase the risk of catheter-related thrombosis in hematology patients: a prospective study. *J Clin Oncol,* 2005, 23(12), 2655-60.

[58] Pronovost, P; Needham, D; Berenholtz, S; Sinopoli, D; Chu, H; Cosgrove, S; et al. An intervention to decrease catheter-related bloodstream infections in the ICU. *N Engl J Med*, 2006, 355(26), 2725-32.

[59] Raad, II. Commentary: zero tolerance for catheter-related bloodstream infections: the unnegotiable objective. *Infect Control Hosp Epidemiol*, 2008, 29(10), 951-3.

[60] O'Grady, NP; Alexander, M; Dellinger, EP; Gerberding, JL; Heard, SO; Maki, DG; et al. Guidelines for the prevention of intravascular catheter-related infections. *Infect Control Hosp Epidemiol*, 2002, 23(12), 759-69.

[61] Simon, A; Beutel, K; Hasan, A; Bode U. Evidenz-basierte Empfehlung zur Anwendung dauerhaft implantierter, zentralvenöser Zugänge in der Pädiatrie. Gesellschaft für Pädiatrische Hämatologie udn Onkologie (GPOH). 3rd Edition ed. Bonn, 2008.

[62] Wenzel, RP; Edmond, MB. Team-based prevention of catheter-related infections. *N Engl J Med*, 2006, 355(26), 2781-3.

[63] Boyce, JM; Pittet, D. Guideline for Hand Hygiene in Health-Care Settings: recommendations of the Healthcare Infection Control Practices Advisory Committee and the HICPAC/SHEA/APIC/IDSA Hand Hygiene Task Force. *Infect Control Hosp Epidemiol*, 2002, 23(12 Suppl), S3-40.

[64] Tablan, OC; Anderson, LJ; Besser, R; Bridges, C; Hajjeh, R. *Guidelines for preventing health-care-associated pneumonia*, 2003, recommendations of CDC and the Healthcare Infection Control Practices Advisory Committee. MMWR Recomm Rep, 2004, 53(RR-3):1-36.

[65] Rayani A; Bode U; Habas E; Fleischhack G; Engelhart S; Exner M; et al. Rotavirus infections in paediatric oncology patients: A matched-pairs analysis. *Scand J Gastroenterol*, 2007, 42(1), 81-7.

[66] Gaur, AH; Liu, T; Knapp, KM; Daw, NC; Rao, BN; Neel, MD; et al. Infections in children and young adults with bone malignancies undergoing limb-sparing surgery. *Cancer* 2005, 104(3), 602-10.

[67] Hota, B. Contamination, disinfection, and cross-colonization: are hospital surfaces reservoirs for nosocomial infection? *Clin Infect Dis*, 2004, 39(8), 1182-9.

[68] Rutala, WA; Weber, DJ. Disinfection and sterilization in health care facilities: what clinicians need to know. *Clin Infect Dis*, 2004, 39(5), 702-9.

[69] Tunkel, AR; Sepkowitz, KA. Infections caused by viridans streptococci in patients with neutropenia. *Clin Infect Dis*, 2002, 34(11), 1524-9.

[70] Lehrnbecher, T; Marshall, D; Gao, C; Chanock, SJ. A second look at anorectal infections in cancer patients in a large cancer institute: the success of early intervention with antibiotics and surgery. *Infection*, 2002, 30(5), 272-6.

[71] Kommission für Krankenhaushygiene und Infektionsprävention. Prävention Gefäßkatheter-assoziierter Infektionen - Empfehlung der Kommission für Krankenhaushygiene und Infektionsprävention am Robert Koch-Institut. *Bundesgesundheitsblatt - Gesundheitsforschung - Gesundheitsschutz*, 2002, 25(11), 907-24.

[72] McKee, C; Berkowitz, I; Cosgrove, SE; Bradley, K; Beers, C; Perl, TM; et al. Reduction of catheter-associated bloodstream infections in pediatric patients: experimentation and reality. *Pediatr Crit Care Med*, 2008, 9(1), 40-6.

[73] Worth, LJ; Slavin, MA; Brown, GV; Black, J. Catheter-related bloodstream infections in hematology: time for standardized surveillance? *Cancer*, 2007, 109(7), 1215-26.

[74] Mahieu, LM; De Dooy, JJ; Lenaerts, AE; Ieven, MM; De Muynck, AO. Catheter manipulations and the risk of catheter-associated bloodstream infection in neonatal intensive care unit patients. *J Hosp Infect*, 2001, 48(1), 20-6.

[75] Safdar, N; Fine, JP; Maki, DG. Meta-analysis: methods for diagnosing intravascular device-related bloodstream infection. *Ann Intern Med*, 2005, 142(6), 451-66.

[76] Raad, II; Luna, M; Khalil, SA; Costerton, JW; Lam, C; Bodey, GP. The relationship between the thrombotic and infectious complications of central venous catheters. *Journal of the American Medical Association*, 1994, 271(13), 1014-6.

[77] Simon, A; Bode, U; Lieber, K; Beutel, K; Fleischhack, G. Review and update of the use of Urokinase in the prevention and management of CVAD-related complications in pediatric oncology patients. *American Journal of Infection Control*, 2008, 36(1), 54-8

[78] Dillon, PW; Jones, GR; Bagnall-Reeb, HA; Buckley, JD; Wiener, ES; Haase, GM. Prophylactic urokinase in the management of long-term venous access devices in children: a Children's Oncology Group study. *J Clin Oncol*, 2004, 22(13), 2718-23.

[79] van Rooden, CJ; Schippers, EF; Guiot, HF; Barge, RM; Hovens, MM; van der Meer, FJ; et al. Prevention of coagulase-negative staphylococcal central venous catheter-related infection using urokinase rinses: a randomized double-blind controlled trial in patients with hematologic malignancies. *J Clin Oncol*, 2008, 26(3), 428-33.

[80] Allon, M. Prophylaxis against dialysis catheter-related bacteremia with a novel antimicrobial lock solution. *Clin Infect Dis*, 2003, 36(12), 1539-44.

[81] Betjes, MG; van Agteren, M. Prevention of dialysis catheter-related sepsis with a citrate-taurolidine-containing lock solution. *Nephrol Dial Transplant*, 2004, 19(6), 1546-51.

[82] Jurewitsch, B; Jeejeebhoy, KN. Taurolidine lock: the key to prevention of recurrent catheter-related bloodstream infections. *Clin Nutr*, 2005, 24(3), 462-5.

[83] van de Wetering, MD; Kuijpers, TW; Taminiau, JA; ten Kate, FJ; Caron, HN. Pseudomembranous and neutropenic enterocolitis in pediatric oncology patients. *Support Care Cancer*, 2003, 11(9), 581-6.

[84] Donskey, CJ. Antibiotic regimens and intestinal colonization with antibiotic-resistant gram-negative bacilli. *Clin Infect Dis*, 2006, 43 Suppl 2, S62-9.

[85] Brook, I. Pseudomembranous colitis in children. *J Gastroenterol Hepatol*, 2005, 20(2), 182-6.

[86] McDonald, LC; Killgore, GE; Thompson, A; Owens, RC; Jr.; Kazakova, SV; Sambol, SP; et al. An epidemic, toxin gene-variant strain of Clostridium difficile. *N Engl J Med* 2005, 353(23), 2433-41.

[87] Bartlett, JG; Perl, TM. The new Clostridium difficile--what does it mean? *N Engl J Med,* 2005, 353(23), 2503-5.

[88] Vonberg, RP; Kuijper, EJ; Wilcox, MH; Barbut, F; Tull, P; Gastmeier, P; et al. Infection control measures to limit the spread of Clostridium difficile. *Clin Microbiol Infect*, 2008, 14 Suppl 5, 2-20.

[89] Nivoix, Y; Velten, M; Letscher-Bru, V; Moghaddam, A; Natarajan-Ame, S; Fohrer, C; et al. Factors associated with overall and attributable mortality in invasive aspergillosis. *Clin Infect Dis*, 2008, 47(9), 1176-84.

[90] Vonberg, RP; Gastmeier, P. Nosocomial aspergillosis in outbreak settings. *J Hosp Infect*, 2006, 63(3), 246-54.

[91] Manuel, RJ; Kibbler, CC. The epidemiology and prevention of invasive aspergillosis. *J Hosp Infect*, 1998, 39(2), 95-109.

[92] Groll, AH; Lehrnbecher, T. New antifungal drugs and the pediatric cancer patient: current status of clinical development. *Klin Padiatr*, 2005, 217(3), 158-68.

[93] Steinbach, WJ. Antifungal agents in children. *Pediatr Clin North Am*, 2005, 52(3), 895-915, viii.

[94] Strasfeld, L; Weinstock, DM. Antifungal prophylaxis among allogeneic hematopoietic stem cell transplant recipients: current issues and new agents. *Expert Rev Anti Infect Ther*, 2006, 4(3), 457-68.

[95] Wisplinghoff, H; Seifert, H; Tallent, SM; Bischoff, T; Wenzel, RP; Edmond, MB. Nosocomial bloodstream infections in pediatric patients in United States hospitals: epidemiology, clinical features and susceptibilities. *Pediatr Infect Dis J*, 2003, 22(8), 686-91.

[96] Paterson, DL, Bonomo, RA. Extended-spectrum beta-lactamases: a clinical update. *Clin Microbiol Rev*, 2005, 18(4), 657-86.

[97] Patel, SJ; Larson, EL; Kubin, CJ; Saiman, L. A review of antimicrobial control strategies in hospitalized and ambulatory pediatric populations. *Pediatr Infect Dis J*, 2007, 26(6), 531-7.

[98] Paterson, DL. The role of antimicrobial management programs in optimizing antibiotic prescribing within hospitals. *Clin Infect Dis*, 2006, 42 Suppl 2, S90-5.

[99] Trampuz, A; Widmer, AF. Infections associated with orthopedic implants. *Curr Opin Infect Dis*, 2006, 19(4), 349-56.

[100] Miller, MA. Clinical management of Clostridium difficile-associated disease. *Clin Infect Dis*, 2007, 45 Suppl 2, S122-8.

[101] Reichenberger, F; Habicht, J; Kaim, A; Dalquen, P; Bernet, F; Schlapfer, R; et al. Lung resection for invasive pulmonary aspergillosis in neutropenic patients with hematologic diseases. *Am J Respir Crit Care Med*, 1998, 158(3), 885-90.

[102] Harbarth, S; Sax, H; Gastmeier, P. The preventable proportion of nosocomial infections: an overview of published reports. *J Hosp Infect*, 2003, 54(4), 258-66, quiz 321.

[103] Larson, E; Nirenberg, A. Evidence-based nursing practice to prevent infection in hospitalized neutropenic patients with cancer. *Oncol Nurs Forum*, 2004, 31(4), 717-25.

[104] McGuckin, M; Shubin, A; Hujcs, M. Interventional patient hygiene model: Infection control and nursing share responsibility for patient safety. *Am J Infect Control*, 2008, 36(1), 59-62.

[105] Chrischilles, EA; Scholz, DA. Dollars and sense: a practical guide to cost analysis for hospital epidemiology and infection control. *Clin Perform Qual Health Care*, 1999, 7(2), 107-11.

[106] Jacobe, SJ; Hassan, A; Veys, P; Mok, Q. Outcome of children requiring admission to an intensive care unit after bone marrow transplantation. *Crit Care Med*, 2003, 31(5), 1299-305.

[107] Holzel, H; de Saxe, M. Septicaemia in paediatric intensive-care patients at the Hospital for Sick Children, Great Ormond Street. *J Hosp Infect*, 1992, 22(3), 185-95.

[108] Coffin, SE; Zaoutis, TE. Infection control, hospital epidemiology, and patient safety. *Infect Dis Clin North Am*, 2005, 19(3), 647-65.

[109] Yokoe, DS; Classen, D. Improving Patient Safety Through Infection Control: A New Healthcare Imperative. Infect Control Hosp Epidemiol 2008, 29(Suppl. 1), S3-S11.

[110] Zell, BL; Goldmann, DA. Healthcare-associated infection and antimicrobial resistance: moving beyond description to prevention. *Infect Control Hosp Epidemiol*, 2007, 28(3), 261-4.

In: Cross Infections: Types, Causes and Prevention
Editors: Jin Dong and Xun Liang

ISBN: 978-1-60741-467-4
© 2009 Nova Science Publishers, Inc.

Chapter V

Prevention of Cross-Transmission of Respiratory Viral Pathogens in Pediatric Oncology Patients

Arne Simon*
Children's Hospital Medical Center University of Bonn, Germany

Introduction

In pediatric patients with cancer and intensive chemotherapy viral infections of the respiratory tract (VRTI) may result in life-threatening complications, including infection of the lower respiratory tract (bronchiolitis, pneumonia, acute respiratory failure). Respiratory tract infection of the upper airways may severely compromise breathing (acute airway obstruction) and cause recurrent aspiration in children with brain tumors, with impaired ability to swallow or with a tracheostoma in place.

As a consequence of the chemotherapy-induced suppression of the cellular and the humoral immune response or of the serious immunodeficiency related to the underlying disease (e.g. leukemia, Hodgkin disease) pediatric cancer patients face an increased risk of hematogenous spread of certain viral pathogens from the respiratory tract to other organs as the liver, the bone-marrow and the central nervous system. In addition, atypical manifestations of viral infections in patients, who are not able to mount a sufficient immune response, may prevent an early recognition of the viral etiology of clinical symptoms and in inadequate treatment due to delayed diagnosis [1].

In a recent study performed in 4 Finnish University Hospitals, Koskenvuo et al. [2] investigated the concomitant presence of 16 viral pathogens in pediatric leukemia patients with blood stream infection (BSI). The prospective evaluation of 156 febrile episodes in 51 children yielded 19 BSI (11%). In 11 of these events (58%) evidence was found for probable

* Corresponding Author: Priv. Doz. Dr. med. Arne Simon Children's Hospital Medical Center University of Bonn Adenauerallee 119, 53113 Bonn, Germany Tel +49-22828733254 Fax +49-22828733301 Email asimon@ukb.uni-bonn.de

concomitant viral infection (5 rhinovirus, 4 respiratory syncytial virus, 2 calicivirus, one enterovirus and one HHV-6 infection). In a previous study from Turku, Finland, microbiologically confirmed respiratory virus infections were found in 28 of 75 (37%) consecutive febrile episodes in 32 children during anticancer treatment [3]. In this clinical setting, viral infection may per se cause severe clinical symptoms or may pave the way for bacterial infections like pneumonia or BSI [4, 5].

From these studies it can be concluded that there is a diagnostic gap considering viral etiologies in pediatric cancer patients with 'fever of unknown origin' due to insufficient efforts to diagnose these events in clinical practice.

The epidemiology and treatment of viral respiratory tract infections in patients, who have received a stem cell transplant, has recently been extensively reviewed in excellent articles [6-9]. This chapter focuses on the prevention of cross transmission of respiratory viral pathogens in pediatric cancer patients with conventional chemotherapy.

Modes of Transmission and Prevention of Patient-To-Patient Transmission

Most pathounLatest video shot of infosys girl www. http://yahoo.com/ gens involved in VRTI are communicable pathogens, which can easily be transmitted from patient to patient. Hand hygiene with a hospital grade hand disinfectant is the most important measure [10] and has to be supplemented with contact, droplet or airborne precautions (Table 1) depending on the mode of transmission of the suspected or confirmed pathogen [11, 12].

It is of utmost importance to educate the patients and their families in the basic principles of hand hygiene as soon as possible during their first admission. Handouts should be used in addition to personal education and should be translated to the patients' native language in case of any difficulties of understanding. Patients and their caregivers and visitors should avoid shaking hands and use disinfectants (in small children only under direct supervision) for hand hygiene in the hospital or the outpatient department, too.

Barrier precautions to prevent patient-to-patient and patient-to-healthcare worker transmission have to be strictly implemented in pediatric hematology and oncology units and in the outpatient department (Table 1).

Most of the viral pathogens involved in VRTI are capable of surviving days or even weeks on contaminated surfaces, toys or items necessary for medical patient care [13].

Stethoscopes have been suspected to be involved in patient to patient transmission of RSV [14] and should be disinfected after each patient contact.

The preventive concept of the unit should include a strategy of regular surface disinfection and disinfection or sterilization of medical products, which are used consequently in more than one patient [15, 16]. Keyboards of notebooks or the consol terminals of other electronic playing devices (e.g. Playstation™), which are often used to alleviate the negative psychosocial impact of hospitalization in particular in adolescent patients, should be disinfected before they are handed out from one patient to the next [17, 18].

In general, visitors are welcome in pediatric oncology departments. Nonetheless, the patients and their families have to be informed, that in any case of respiratory tract infection, fever or rash, symptomatic friends and relatives should refrain from visiting the unit.

Table 1. Mode of transmission, prevention (in addition to standard hygiene precautions and isolation) and immunization options

Virus	Mode of transmission	Prevention [10-12, 96]	Immunisation
Measles* VZV (Chickenpox)* (Influenza)*#	Airborne	FFP 2 mask plus droplet* precautions plus contact precautions	Health care workers should be - immune or immunized against measles, VZV - immunized against influenza (yearly) Passive immunization (patients after contact): Measles: standard immunoglobulin VZV: VZV hyperimmunoglobulin¢
Influenza virus Respiratory syncytial virus Human Metapneumovirus Parainfluenzavirus Enterovirus RTI ADV RTI Human Bocavirus (?)+	Droplets	Droplet precautions surgical masks, gowns, gloves Eye protection in outbreak situations (RSV)	Palivizumab available but not licensed for prevention of RSV infection in immunocompromized children (no controlled data available).
VZV (zoster, shingles) Cytomegalovirus Human Bocavirus (?)+	Direct contact Saliva shedding Fecal-oral?	Contact precautions	Health care workers should be - immune or immunized against VZV

RTI = respirator tract infection; GIT = gastrointestinal infection; RSV = Respiratory syncytial virus VZV = Varicella zoster virus ADV = adenovirus

Still a matter of debate. Please refer to [97-99]

¢ Some institutions prefer the prophylactic administration of acyclovir (see text)

‡ Use specific hand disinfectant with high ethanol content [24]

The rate of Latest video shot of infosys girl www.http://yahoo.com/ control program has recently been investigated by Gomez-Villa et al. [19] during 4 winter seasons. The rate of nosocomial viral respiratory infection decreased from 6.09 episodes per 100 patients admitted during the first study year to 1.46 episodes per 100 patients admitted during the last study year. Although this study was performed in a toddler ward, the results should encourage pediatric oncologists to implement an approach of early diagnostic efforts [20] and subsequent isolation in pediatric cancer units too [21]. Diagnostic methods to confirm the etiology of an acute VRTI are listed in Table 2.

Table 2 Diagnostic tools and clinical manifestation of respiratory viral infections

Virus (Family) DNA vs. RNA Virus	Diagnostic tools	Clinical manifestation
Adenovirus (Adenoviridae) DNA Virus	AT, CC, PCR, qPCR	Pneumonia, hepatitis, gastroenteritis, hemorrhagic cystitis
Cytomegalovirus (Herpesviridae) DNA Virus	CC, SVT, pp65 AT PCR, qPCR Serology [IgG, IgM] TB (lung, oesophagus, colon)	interstitial pneumonia hepatitis, oesophagitis, enterocolitis retinitis
Enterovirus (Enteroviridae) RNA Virus	Rt-PCR, qPCR, CC	Gastroenteritis, respiratory tract infections, gastroenteritis
Human Bocavirus (Parvoviridae) DNA Virus	PCR, NASBA	Lower respiratory tract infection? disseminated viral infection?
Human Metapneumovirus (Paramyxoviridae) RNA Virus	Rt-PCR, CC, AT, SVT, IF	Bronchitis, pneumonia
Influenzavirus (Orthomyxoviridae) RNA Virus	Rt-PCR, CC, AT, SVT, IF	Croup syndrom, bronchitis, pneumonia
Measles virus (Paramyxoviridae) RNA Virus	Rt-PCRCC, SVT Serology [IgG, IgM]	Measles, tracheitis, giant cell pneumonia Measles-associated encephalopathy
Parainfluenzavirus (Paramyxoviridae) RNA Virus	AT, IF, SVT Rt-PCR	Croup Syndrom, Bronchitis, Pneumonia
Respiratory Syncytial Virus (Paramycoviridae) RNA Virus	AT, IF, CC, SVT, Rt-PCR	Croup Syndrom, bronchitis, pneumonia
Varizella zoster virus (Herpesviridae) DNA Virus	PCR Serology [IgG, IgM] (TB)	Chickenpox, disseminated varicella with multiorgan involvement, pneumonitis, hepatitis, encephalitis, cerebellitis shingles (zoster)

Commercially available antigen tests for norovirus yield too many false positive results.

§ For details refer to the text.

AT = Antigen testing

IF = Immune fluorescence

CC = Cell culture

TB = tissue biopsy with immunologic staining

PCR = Polymerase chain reaction

qPCR = Polymerase chain reaction = quantitiave PCR (defining viral loads)

rt-PCR = reverse transcipatse-Polymerase chain reaction (for RNA viruses)

qrt-PCR = quantitiave rt-PCR (defining viral loads)

SVT shell vial technique (viral antigens are detected in the supernant of cell culture)

Prolonged Viral Shedding

Prolonged symptomatic [22, 23] and asymptomatic [21, 24, 25] shedding of contagious virus particles is often observed in immunocompromized children. This phenomenon may last weeks or month and contributes significantly to the risk of nosocomial transmission.

Pediatric patients, who continue to shed contagious viruses in respiratory secretions, urine or stool after cessation of clinical symptoms, have to be separated from other immunocompromized patients by contact or droplet isolation as long as the viral shedding persists (see Table 1). Thus, in the conception of inpatient care facilities for pediatric oncology patients at least 30% of all rooms for patient care have to be attributed to the isolation of patients infected or colonized with communicable pathogens [26].

Rhinovirus and Enterovirus

Enteroviruses, small RNA viruses, include coxsackie viruses A and B, echoviruses, enteroviruses 68-71 and polioviruses. Enteroviridae replicate in the gastrointestinal tract; their transmission occurs predominantly by the fecal-oral route.

Enterovirus infection may be accompanied or followed by a meningitis, which follows a benign clinical course in most cases or an encephalitis [27] that includes a clinical spectrum from altered mental status to coma, and my be associated with long-term neurologic sequelae. On the one hand, the clinical significance of a positive rhinovirus or enterovirus PCR from respiratory specimens is uncertain, because after the onset of symptomatic respiratory infection enterovirus RNA may take 2-3 weeks and rhinovirus RNA 5-6 weeks to disappear from nasal mucus [28].

On the other hand, chronic persistence of replicating rhinovirus in the lung with fatal outcome has been reported in lung transplant recipients [29] and severe lower respiratory tract infections have been attributed to rhinovirus infections in some prospective case series [2, 3, 30]. One study from Greece investigated the clinical presentation, severity and outcome of EV infections in pediatric cancer patients [31]. Samples of whole blood, throat swab, cerebrospinal fluid (CSF), bone marrow and urine underwent EV genome amplification by RT-PCR and nucleotide sequencing. EV infection was confirmed in 55 of 104 evaluated patients.

Encephalitis was diagnosed in 10%, myocardial involvement and hemophagocytosis were observed in 5%, respectively. Most children with EV-infection had acute lymphoblastic leukemia or lymphoma. The fatality rate was 14.5% (n=8).

Although controlled studies are missing, experiences in patients with congenital agammaglobulinemia and case reports suggest, that high dose (2g/kg) IVIG treatment may be beneficial in immunocompromized patients with EV infection [31]. Pleconaril, which inhibits the replication of pircornaviruses, has recently become available for clinical use [32]. Pleconaril should be administered in an early stage of severe EV infection to prevent multiorgan failure. Prospective studies in children with cancer are still not available [33, 34].

Influenzavirus

Influenza virus infection may cause acute respiratory failure and death in immunocompromized patients [35]. Distinguishing influenza from bacterial infection is extremely difficult in pediatric cancer patients with subtle clinical signs of respiratory tract infection and with high fever as the leading symptom. Typical complaints in adolescents and adults, as headache, myalgia, fatigue and dizziness are difficult to determine in young children. Influenzavirus infection may be accompanied or followed by bacterial pneumonia (e.g. *Haemophilus influenzae, Streptococcus pneumoniae, Staphylococcus aureus*) and sepsis [4]. In order to prevent nosocomial spread, NPA specimen from pediatric cancer patients hospitalized with respiratory tract infection during the influenza season should be tested in a timely fashion for influenza A and B virus by PCR-based methods. In addition to the early implementation of barrier precautions (Tab.1), this is advisable from the perspective of early antiviral treatment. The neuraminidase inhibitors, oseltamivir [36] and zanamivir [37] are effective against both influenza A and B viruses [38]; treatment should start at best in the first 48 h ours after the onset of symptoms [39].

Respiratory Syncytial Virus (RSV)

RSV, an RNA virus from the subfamily pneumovirus, family paramyxoviridae, is responsible for up to 70% of all cases of bronchiolitis and 20-50% of all cases of pneumonia in infants and young children [40]. Immunocompromized children face an increased risk of a severe clinical course which may lead to acute respirator failure and death. El Saleeby et al. [41] identified profound lymphopenia, with absolute lymphocyte counts of $< 0.1 \times 10^9/l$, and age of ≤ 2 years as significant risk factors for severe disease in 58 RSV infected pediatric cancer patients. In this study, the overall mortality rate was 8.6%.

RSV-infected patients should be kept in droplet isolation according to fixed local standards of hygiene [42]. The disinfection of hands [10], use of gowns, masks and disposable gloves in contact with patients and possibly contaminated surfaces are essential. In 25 of 39 (64%) patients with RSV infection from our institution, the next chemotherapy had to be postponed due to the RSV-infection. This may result in decreased dose intensity with a negative impact on the treatment perspective for the underlying malignancy.

Therapy for RSV-infection is symptomatic (adequate fluid intake, treatment of fever, monitoring, oxygen supplementation and, if necessary, mask-CPAP or mechanical ventilation). Corticosteroids should be avoided; salbutamol (albuterol) and epinephrine inhalations should only be used in patients who show an objective clinical response. Although secondary bacterial infections in RSV-infected healthy children are rare (<5%), standard empirical antibacterial treatment is recommended in cancer patients with febrile neutropenia and RSV infection.

Mainly due to safety and compliance issues and to technical difficulties it is not feasible to treat non-intubated infants and young children with ribavirin inhalation delivered at a concentration of 20mg/mL for 18 hours via a small particle aerosol generator unit and administered via a face mask inside a scavenging tent to prevent environmental contamination' [9, 43]. In addition, the objective benefit of this intervention is still under debate [44].

In patients with severe pneumonia due to RSV-infection, intravenous administration of ribavirin may be an option [45]. There is still no evidence-based treatment algorithm available for patients outside the acute phase of allogeneic stem cell transplantation. Thus, the decision to treat a symptomatic patient with confirmed RSV infection with ribavirin has to be made on an individual basis. In our unit, we use ribavirin (p.o., iv.) only in patients with progressive respiratory failure or in AML patients during induction treatment.

Standard immunoglobulin provides no protection because the resulting antibody titers are not sufficient. Passive immunoprophylaxis with humanized monoclonal antibodies against the F-protein of the virus (palivizumab) has not been investigated in pediatric cancer patients [46, 47]. Although Chávez-Bueno et al. [48] reported favorable preliminary data on combination treatment (ribavirin and iv palivizumab), de Fontbrune et al. [49] could not demonstrate a significant impact of palivizumab on the clinical course and survival of 19 allogenic stem cell transplant recipients with RSV-infection. Considering the very limited options for highly immunocompromized patients [43, 50], a prospective randomized multicenter study with motavizumab, an ultra-potent, affinity-matured, humanized monoclonal antibody [51] should be debated in pediatric cancer patients with severe RSV-infection [52].

Human Metapneumovirus (hMPV)

The human Metapneumovirus, an RNA virus from the subfamily pneumovirus, family paramyxoviridae, was first identified in 2001 in the nasopharyngeal aspirates of young children from the Netherlands with respiratory tract illness [53].

The symptoms of hMPV infection do not differ significantly from the clinical picture of other viral RTI [54]. Clinical severity has been described to be comparable to RSV infection [55]. HMPV has been detected in immunocompromized patients with severe lower RTI. In 2002, Pelletier et al. [56] described the clinical course of a girl with acute lymphoblastic leukemia who experienced two episodes of hMPV infection at the age of 7 months and again at 17 months while still receiving cytotoxic chemotherapy. While the first infection was an episode of febrile neutropenia without severe complications, the second hMPV infection resulted in acute respiratory failure and death. We cared for a 10-month-old infant with rhabdomyosarcoma who experienced an hMPV infection while receiving intensive induction chemotherapy. The febrile neutropenic patient received Piperacillin-Tazobactam and Teicoplanin intravenously and no pathogen other than hMPV was detected in respiratory, blood and urine cultures. The fever subsided and the patient recovered uneventfully when the neutrophil count increased above $1 \times 10^9/l$ again. In a recent study, 3% of transplant patients (5 out of 163) with pneumonia were found to be hMPV-infected. Four of these patients died of respiratory insufficiency within 40 days after transplantation (in three of these only hMPV was detected). All these patients had severe lymphopenia [57]. Currently no established treatment for hMPV infections exists. Intravenous ribavirin may be considered in mechanically ventilated hMPV infected patients with acute respiratory failure [45] since ribavirin shows antiviral activity in vitro [58, 59].

Human Bocavirus (HBOV)

Human Bocavirus is a recently identified member of the parvoviridae family [60] and most probably represents the second parvovirus responsible for diseases in humans [61, 62]. This clinical spectrum is in accordance with other viral acute RTIs, similar to the situation in RSV infections [63] and in HMPV infections [55, 64]. There are no distinct clinical signs to aid the medical practitioner in differentiating HBoV infection from that associated with other viruses on clinical grounds alone [65, 66]. Many case series suggest that HBoV may cause central pneumonia as well as interstitial and lobar pneumonia especially in newborns and infants.

As in many other viral respiratory tract pathogens both, clinical symptoms, laboratory parameters and radiological findings are not sufficiently specific to make a clear distinction between a bacterial or viral cause of pneumonia [65, 67-70]. Symptoms seem to persist for 1-2 weeks on average [71, 72]. Several clinical research groups have reported HBoV-positive immunocompromized patients [73-75]. Arnold and co-workers described 2 pediatric patients positive for HBoV after organ transplantation [73]. Kupfer et al. have recently published the clinical case of a severe infection in a 28 year-old HBoV-positive female patient with malignant B-cell lymphoma [76]. Schenk et al. recently described a disseminated HBoV infection in a 4.5 year old child after allogeneic stem cell transplantation [77]

Gastrointestinal symptoms have been described in up to 25% of all patients [73, 78, 79]. Further studies in immunocompromized pediatric patients should include the testing of stool samples for HBoV to confirm viral shedding, and broader investigation of a possible role for HBoV as an enteric pathogen. Since other members of the parvoviridae are definitely known to be highly resistant to disinfectants [80, 81] such investigations should be done for HBoV, too [61].

Varicella Zoster Virus

Varicella zoster virus (VZV) infection may be accompanied or followed by viral pneumonitis in pediatric cancer patients. Diagnosing disseminated VZV infection with visceral involvement is often difficult in immunocompromized patients due to atypical clinical presentation with few or no skin lesions and severe abdominal or back pain [82]. Prompt initiation of empirical treatment with acyclovir pending results of PCR for VZV from skin lesions or serum samples is warranted in this clinical setting [83]. The role of VZIG in prophylaxis and treatment is still debated in severely immunocompromized children and adolescents [82]. In our unit, children with cancer and conventional chemotherapy receive prophylactic acyclovir from day 7 after exposure for 7 days (1200mg/m^2/day p.o.) [84] Close clinical follow up investigations are ensured in these patients. If a breakthrough VZV infection occurs, the child is immediately hospitalized and treated with acyclovir intravenously. Although this approach has now been successfully followed by us for more than 10 years, no randomized controlled study has been published yet confirming the efficacy and safety of this regimen in pediatric cancer patients. The most controversial issue of debate in such a study will be the definition of a relevant event of exposure in severely immunocompromized children [82].

A retrospective case series from the Children's Hospital of Pittsburgh [85] revealed that 49% of 41 children with VZV-infection during treatment for acute lymphoblastic leukemia had received prophylaxis with varicella zoster immunoglobulin (VZIG). Twenty-nine of the 42 cases (70%) had disease limited to the skin.

Thirteen cases (30%) had extracutaneous involvement, and five of these episodes (12% of all cases) ended in death. Risk factors for progressive varicella included age greater than 6 years and intensive immunosuppressive therapy at the time of exposure. Six of eight patients with progressive varicella, including two who died, had received VZIG. The clinical presentation in 10 of 13 patients with progressive disease and in four of five patients who died was dominated by severe abdominal and/or back pain. In seven cases, these symptoms preceded the development of skin lesions by several days, and in six patients were associated with extensive involvement of the spleen by varicella, as demonstrated by the presence of Howell-Jolly bodies on peripheral-blood smear. No patient with uncomplicated VZV infection was reported to have had premonitory pain.

Hill et al. [86] examined the relationship between steroid therapy for ALL and severity of VZV infection in 697 children with ALL. Of these, 110 (15.8%) developed primary VZV infection. Of the patients whose VZV infection was diagnosed within 3 weeks of receipt of prednisone, 70% had severe infection, whereas only 44% of those who had not received prednisone within 3 weeks had severe infection (odds ratio 2.9; CI_{95}: 1.1-7.9). By multivariate analysis, older age at ALL diagnosis, years from ALL diagnosis to VZV diagnosis, and VZV diagnosis during or within 3 weeks of prednisone therapy all were independently associated with an increased risk for severe infection.

Immunization of Health Care Workers, Attending Physicians and Relatives

Medical personnel (health care workers, physicians, and physiotherapists) involved in clinical care of immunocompromized patients should be immune or immunized against measles [87, 88] and varicella [89, 90] and should participate in the yearly influenza immunization campaign [91-94]. This should be the case for all members of the patient's family, too, to improve herd immunity. Since vaccine-associated rashes after measles and varicella immunization in healthy family members of immunocompromized children are uncommon and mild, it is likely that transmission of vaccine virus will also be uncommon [95]. The theoretical possibility of transmission of attenuated vaccine-virus isolates in household contacts does not result in a contraindication for the immunization of non-immune healthy household members against measles and varicella. When a vaccine associated rash occurs in a family member, preventive administration of standard immunoglobulin (measles) or acyclovir (varicella) to the patient should be considered during intensive treatment periods.

Conclusion

Physicians attending pediatric cancer patients during intensive conventional anticancer treatment have to be aware of the potential pathogens of viral respiratory tract infection, their mode of transmission and the best diagnostic approach to detect viral infections in this high risk population as timely as possible.

Pediatric cancer units should implement a comprehensive preventive strategy to avoid cross transmission, including a good practice of hand disinfection (physicians, health care workers and even patients and their families), isolation and cohortation of infected patients for the duration of viral shedding with adequate barrier precautions, as well as regular disinfection of hand contact surfaces and medical products and regular immunization of healthcare workers and other caregivers.

Newly detected, emerging viral pathogens, as HMPV or HBoV may be recognized as a threat to severely immunocompromized pediatric cancer patients too, but there is still a lack of knowledge considering their nosocomial epidemiology. More studies considering the efficacy, feasibility and the cost of prospectively evaluated concepts to prevent cross transmission of viral respiratory pathogens are needed in pediatric oncology patients.

References

[1] Simon, A; Schildgen, O; Schuster, F. Viral infections in children with cancer. *Arch Dis Child*, 2008.

[2] Koskenvuo, M; Mottonen, M; Rahiala, J; Saarinen-Pihkala, UM; Riikonen, P; Waris, M; et al. Mixed bacterial-viral infections in septic children with leukemia. *Pediatr Infect Dis J*, 2007, 26(12), 1133-6.

[3] Arola, M; Ruuskanen, O; Ziegler, T; Salmi, TT. Respiratory virus infections during anticancer treatment in children. *Pediatr Infect Dis J*, 1995, 14(8), 690-4.

[4] Peltola, V; Waris, M; Hyypia, T; Ruuskanen, O. Respiratory viruses in children with invasive pneumococcal disease. *Clin Infect Dis*, 2006, 43(2), 266-8.

[5] Lowenthal, A; Livni, G; Amir, J; Samra, Z; Ashkenazi, S. Secondary bacteremia after rotavirus gastroenteritis in infancy. *Pediatrics*, 2006, 117(1), 224-6.

[6] Lee, I; Barton, TD. Viral respiratory tract infections in transplant patients: epidemiology, recognition and management. *Drugs*, 2007, 67(10), 1411-27.

[7] Ison, MG. Respiratory viral infections in transplant recipients. *Antivir Ther*, 2007, 12(4 Pt B), 627-38.

[8] Kim, YJ; Boeckh, M; Englund, JA. Community respiratory virus infections in immunocompromised patients: hematopoietic stem cell and solid organ transplant recipients, and individuals with human immunodeficiency virus infection. *Semin Respir Crit Care Med*, 2007, 28(2), 222-42.

[9] Hicks, KL; Chemaly, RF; Kontoyiannis, DP. Common community respiratory viruses in patients with cancer: more than just "common colds". *Cancer*, 2003, 97(10), 2576-87.

[10] Boyce, JM; Pittet, D. Guideline for Hand Hygiene in Health-Care Settings: recommendations of the Healthcare Infection Control Practices Advisory Committee and the HICPAC/SHEA/APIC/IDSA Hand Hygiene Task Force. *Infect Control Hosp Epidemiol*, 2002, 23(12 Suppl), S3-40.

[11] Garner, JS. Guideline for isolation precautions in hospitals. Part I. Evolution of isolation practices, Hospital Infection Control Practices Advisory Committee. *Am J Infect Control*, 1996, 24(1), 24-31.

[12] Garner, JS. Guideline for isolation precautions in hospitals. The Hospital Infection Control Practices Advisory Committee. *Infect Control Hosp Epidemiol*, 1996, 17(1), 53-80.

[13] Kramer, A; Schwebke, I; Kampf, G. How long do nosocomial pathogens persist on inanimate surfaces? A systematic review. *BMC Infect Dis*, 2006, 6(1), 130.

[14] Blydt-Hansen, T; Subbarao, K; Quennec, P; McDonald, J. Recovery of respiratory syncytial virus from stethoscopes by conventional viral culture and polymerase chain reaction. *Pediatr Infect Dis J*, 1999, 18(2), 164-5.

[15] Rutala, WA; Weber, DJ. Disinfection and sterilization in health care facilities: what clinicians need to know. *Clin Infect Dis*, 2004, 39(5), 702-9.

[16] Hota, B. Contamination, disinfection, and cross-colonization: are hospital surfaces reservoirs for nosocomial infection? *Clin Infect Dis*, 2004, 39(8), 1182-9.

[17] Neely, AN; Maley, MP. Dealing with contaminated computer keyboards and microbial survival. *Am J Infect Control*, 2001, 29(2), 131-2.

[18] Neely, AN; Sittig, DF. Basic microbiologic and infection control information to reduce the potential transmission of pathogens to patients via computer hardware. *J Am Med Inform Assoc*, 2002, 9(5), 500-8.

[19] Gomez-Villa, RJ; Comas-Garcia, A; Lopez-Rojas, V; Perez-Gonzalez, LF; Sanchez-Alvarado, J; Salazar-Zaragoza R; et al. Effect of an infection control program on the frequency of nosocomial viral respiratory infections. *Infect Control Hosp Epidemiol*, 2008, 29(6), 556-8.

[20] Barenfanger, J; Drake, C; Leon, N; Mueller, T; Troutt, T. Clinical and financial benefits of rapid detection of respiratory viruses: an outcomes study. *J Clin Microbiol*, 2000, 38(8), 2824-8.

[21] Simon, A; Khurana, K; Wilkesmann, A; Muller, A; Engelhart, S; Exner, M; et al. Nosocomial respiratory syncytial virus infection: Impact of prospective surveillance and targeted infection control. *Int J Hyg Environ Health*, 2006, 209(4), 317-24.

[22] Lee, BE; Pang, XL; Robinson, JL; Bigam, D; Monroe, SS; Preiksaitis, JK. Chronic Norovirus and Adenovirus Infection in a Solid Organ Transplant Recipient. *Pediatr Infect Dis J*, 2008.

[23] Blanchard, SS; Gerrek, M, Siegel, C, Czinn, SJ. Significant morbidity associated with RSV infection in immunosuppressed children following liver transplantation: case report and discussion regarding need of routine prophylaxis. *Pediatr Transplant*, 2006, 10(7), 826-9.

[24] Simon, A; Schildgen, O; Maria Eis-Hubinger, A; Hasan, C; Bode, U; Buderus, S; et al. Norovirus outbreak in a pediatric oncology unit. *Scand J Gastroenterol*, 2006, 41(6), 693-9.

[25] Rayani, A; Bode, U; Habas, E; Fleischhack, G; Engelhart, S; Exner, M; et al. Rotavirus infections in paediatric oncology patients: A matched-pairs analysis. *Scand J Gastroenterol*, 2007, 42(1), 81-7.

[26] Langley, JM; Hanakowski, M; Bortolussi, R. Demand for isolation beds in a pediatric hospital. *Am J Infect Control*, 1994, 22(4), 207-11.

[27] Frange, P; Michon, J; Fromantin, I; Franck, N; Safar, E; Escande, MC; et al. Enterovirus 71 meningoencephalitis during chemotherapy in a child with metastatic osteosarcoma. *J Pediatr Hematol Oncol*, 2007, 29(8), 566-8.
[28] Jartti, T; Lehtinen, P; Vuorinen, T; Koskenvuo, M; Ruuskanen, O. Persistence of rhinovirus and enterovirus RNA after acute respiratory illness in children. *J Med Virol*, 2004, 72(4), 695-9.
[29] Kaiser L; Aubert JD; Pache JC; Deffernez, C; Rochat, T; Garbino, J; et al. Chronic rhinoviral infection in lung transplant recipients. *Am J Respir Crit Care Med*, 2006, 174(12), 1392-9.
[30] Christensen, MS; Nielsen, LP; Hasle, H. Few but severe viral infections in children with cancer: A prospective RT-PCR and PCR-based 12-month study. *Pediatr Blood Cancer*, 2005.
[31] Moschovi, MA; Katsibardi, K; Theodoridou, M; Michos, AG; Tsakris, A; Spanakis, N; et al. Enteroviral infections in children with malignant disease: a 5-year study in a single institution. *J Infect*, 2007, 54(4), 387-92.
[32] Rotbart, HA; Webster, AD. Treatment of potentially life-threatening enterovirus infections with pleconaril. *Clin Infect Dis*, 2001, 32(2), 228-35.
[33] Desmond, RA; Accortt, NA; Talley, L; Villano, SA; Soong, SJ; Whitley, RJ. Enteroviral meningitis: natural history and outcome of pleconaril therapy. *Antimicrob Agents Chemother*, 2006, 50(7), 2409-14.
[34] Barnard, DL. Current status of anti-picornavirus therapies. *Curr Pharm Des*, 2006, 12(11), 1379-90.
[35] Heikkinen, T. Influenza in children. *Acta Paediatr*, 2006, 95(7), 778-84.
[36] Whitley, RJ; Hayden, FG; Reisinger, KS; Young, N; Dutkowski, R; Ipe, D; et al. Oral oseltamivir treatment of influenza in children. *Pediatr Infect Dis J*, 2001, 20(2), 127-33.
[37] Hedrick, JA; Barzilai, A; Behre, U; Henderson, FW; Hammond, J; Reilly, L; et al. Zanamivir for treatment of symptomatic influenza A and B infection in children five to twelve years of age: a randomized controlled trial. *Pediatr Infect Dis J*, 2000, 19(5), 410-7.
[38] Cooper, NJ; Sutton, AJ; Abrams, KR; Wailoo, A; Turner, D; Nicholson, KG. Effectiveness of neuraminidase inhibitors in treatment and prevention of influenza A and B: systematic review and meta-analyses of randomised controlled trials. *Bmj*, 2003, 326(7401), 1235.
[39] Chemaly, RF; Torres, HA; Aguilera, EA; Mattiuzzi, G; Cabanillas, M; Kantarjian, H; et al. Neuraminidase inhibitors improve outcome of patients with leukemia and influenza: an observational study. *Clin Infect Dis*, 2007, 44(7), 964-7.
[40] Black, CP. Systematic review of the biology and medical management of respiratory syncytial virus infection. *Respir Care*, 2003, 48(3), 209-31; discussion 31-3.
[41] Saleeby, El; Somes, CM; DeVincenzo, GW; Gaur, JP; Risk, AH. factors for severe respiratory syncytial virus disease in children with cancer: *the importance of lymphopenia and young age. Pediatrics*, 2008, 121(2), 235-43.
[42] Taylor, GS; Vipond, IB; Caul, EO. Molecular epidemiology of outbreak of respiratory syncytial virus within bone marrow transplantation unit. *J Clin Microbiol*, 2001, 39(2), 801-3.

[43] Hirsch, HH; Steffen, I; Francioli, P; Widmer, AF. [Respiratory syncytial virus infections: measures in immunocompromised patients]. *Schweiz Rundsch Med Prax*, 2006, 95(3), 61-6.

[44] Boeckh, M; Englund, J; Li, Y; Miller, C; Cross, A; Fernandez, H; et al. Randomized controlled multicenter trial of aerosolized ribavirin for respiratory syncytial virus upper respiratory tract infection in hematopoietic cell transplant recipients. *Clin Infect Dis*, 2007, 44(2), 245-9.

[45] Raza, K; Ismailjee, SB; Crespo, M; Studer, SM; Sanghavi, S; Paterson, DL; et al. Successful outcome of human metapneumovirus (hMPV) pneumonia in a lung transplant recipient treated with intravenous ribavirin. *J Heart Lung Transplant*, 2007, 26(8), 862-4.

[46] Simoes, EA; Groothuis, JR. Respiratory syncytial virus prophylaxis--the story so far. *Respir Med*, 2002, 96 Suppl B:S15-24.

[47] Khanna, N; Widmer, AF; Decker, M; Steffen, I; Halter, J; Heim, D; et al. Respiratory syncytial virus infection in patients with hematological diseases: single-center study and review of the literature. *Clin Infect Dis*, 2008, 46(3), 402-12.

[48] Chavez-Bueno, S; Mejias, A; Merryman, RA; Ahmad, N; Jafri, HS; Ramilo, O. Intravenous palivizumab and ribavirin combination for respiratory syncytial virus disease in high-risk pediatric patients. *Pediatr Infect Dis J*, 2007, 26(12), 1089-93.

[49] de Fontbrune, FS; Robin, M; Porcher, R; Scieux, C; de Latour, RP; Ferry, C; et al. Palivizumab treatment of respiratory syncytial virus infection after allogeneic hematopoietic stem cell transplantation. *Clin Infect Dis*, 2007, 45(8), 1019-24.

[50] Whimbey, E; Champlin, RE; Englund, JA; Mirza, NQ; Piedra, PA; Goodrich, JM; et al. Combination therapy with aerosolized ribavirin and intravenous immunoglobulin for respiratory syncytial virus disease in adult bone marrow transplant recipients. *Bone Marrow Transplant*, 1995, 16(3), 393-9.

[51] Wu, H; Pfarr, DS; Johnson, S; Brewah, YA; Woods, RM; Patel, NK; et al. Development of motavizumab, an ultra-potent antibody for the prevention of respiratory syncytial virus infection in the upper and lower respiratory tract. *J Mol Biol*, 2007, 368(3), 652-65.

[52] Simon, A; Schildgen, O; Panning, M; Bode, U; Eis-Hubinger, A. RSV-infection in patients with cancer – still more questions than answers. *Clin Infect Dis*, 2008, 46(15 June), 1933-4.

[53] van den Hoogen, BG; de Jong, JC; Groen, J, Kuiken, T; de Groot, R; Fouchier, RA; et al. A newly discovered human pneumovirus isolated from young children with respiratory tract disease. *Nat Med*, 2001, 7(6), 719-24.

[54] Schildgen, O; Simon, A; Wilkesmann, A; Williams, JV; Eis-Hubinger, AM; Roggendorf, M; et al. The human metapneumovirus (HMPV): biology, epidemiological features, and clinical characteristics of infection. *Reviews in Medical Microbiology*, 2006, 17(1), 11-25.

[55] Wilkesmann, A; Schildgen, O; Eis-Hubinger, AM; Geikowski, T; Glatzel, T; Lentze, MJ; et al. Human metapneumovirus infections cause similar symptoms and clinical severity as respiratory syncytial virus infections. *Eur J Pediatr*, 2006, 165(7), 467-75.

[56] Pelletier, G; Dery, P; Abed, Y; Boivin, G. Respiratory tract reinfections by the new human Metapneumovirus in an immunocompromised child. *Emerg Infect Dis*, 2002, 8(9), 976-8.

[57] Englund, JA; Boeckh, M; Kuypers, J; Nichols, WG; Hackman, RC; Morrow, RA; et al. Brief communication: fatal human metapneumovirus infection in stem-cell transplant recipients. *Ann Intern Med*, 2006, 144(5), 344-9.

[58] Hamelin, ME; Prince, GA; Boivin, G. Effect of ribavirin and glucocorticoid treatment in a mouse model of human metapneumovirus infection. *Antimicrob Agents Chemother*, 2006, 50(2), 774-7.

[59] Wyde, PR; Chetty, SN; Jewell, AM; Boivin, G; Piedra, PA. Comparison of the inhibition of human metapneumovirus and respiratory syncytial virus by ribavirin and immune serum globulin in vitro. *Antiviral Res*, 2003, 60(1), 51-9.

[60] Anderson, LJ. Human bocavirus: a new viral pathogen. *Clin Infect Dis*, 2007, 44(7), 911-2.

[61] Schildgen, O; Muller, A; Allander, T; Mackay, IM; Volz, S; Kupfer, B; et al. Human bocavirus: passenger or pathogen in acute respiratory tract infections? *Clin Microbiol Rev*, 2008, 21(2), 291-304, table of contents.

[62] Volz, S; Schildgen, O; Klinkenberg, D; Ditt, V; Muller, A; Tillmann, RL; et al. Prospective study of Human Bocavirus (HBoV) infection in a pediatric university hospital in Germany 2005/2006. *J Clin Virol*, 2007, 40(3), 229-35.

[63] Weigl, JA; Puppe, W; Schmitt, HJ. Can respiratory syncytial virus etiology be diagnosed clinically? A hospital-based case-control study in children under two years of age. *Eur J Epidemiol*, 2003, 18(5), 431-9.

[64] Williams, JV. The clinical presentation and outcomes of children infected with newly identified respiratory tract viruses. *Infect Dis Clin North Am*, 2005, 19(3), 569-84.

[65] Kleines, M; Scheithauer, S; Rackowitz, A; Ritter, K; Hausler, M. High prevalence of human bocavirus detected in young children with severe acute lower respiratory tract disease using a standard PCR protocol and a novel real time PCR protocol. *J Clin Microbiol*, 2007.

[66] Allander, T; Tammi, MT; Eriksson, M; Bjerkner, A; Tiveljung-Lindell, A; Andersson, B. Cloning of a human parvovirus by molecular screening of respiratory tract samples. *Proc Natl Acad Sci U S A*, 2005, 102(36), 12891-6.

[67] Korppi, M. Community-acquired pneumonia in children: issues in optimizing antibacterial treatment. *Paediatr Drugs*, 2003, 5(12), 821-32.

[68] Korppi, M. Mixed microbial aetiology of community-acquired pneumonia in children. Apmis 2002, 110(7-8), 515-22.

[69] McIntosh K. Community-acquired pneumonia in children. N Engl J Med 2002, 346(6), 429-37.

[70] Fry, AM; Lu, X; Chittaganpitch, M; Peret, T; Fischer, J; Dowell, SF; et al. Human bocavirus: a novel parvovirus epidemiologically associated with pneumonia requiring hospitalization in Thailand. *J Infect Dis*, 2007, 195(7), 1038-45.

[71] Regamey, N; Frey, U; Deffernez, C; Latzin, P; Kaiser, L. Isolation of Human Bocavirus from Swiss Infants with Respiratory Infections. *Pediatr Infect Diṣ J*, 2007, 26(2), 177-9.

[72] Allander, T; Jartti, T; Gupta, S; Niesters, HG; Lehtinen, P; Osterback, R; et al. Human bocavirus and acute wheezing in children. *Clin Infect Dis*, 2007, 44(7), 904-10.

[73] Arnold, JC; Singh, KK; Spector, SA; Sawyer, MH. Human bocavirus: prevalence and clinical spectrum at a children's hospital. *Clin Infect Dis*, 2006, 43(3), 283-8.

[74] Smuts, H; Hardie, D. Human Bocavirus in Hospitalized Children, South Africa. *Emerg Infect Dis*, 2006, 12(9), 1457-8.

[75] Manning, A; Russell, V; Eastick, K; Leadbetter, GH; Hallam, N; Templeton, K; et al. Epidemiological profile and clinical associations of human bocavirus and other human parvoviruses. *J Infect Dis*, 2006, 194(9), 1283-90.

[76] Kupfer, B; Vehreschild, J; Cornely, O; Kaiser, R; Plum, G; Viazov, S; et al. Severe Pneumonia and Human Bocavirus in an Adult. *Emerg Infect Dis*, 2006, 12(10), 1614-6.

[77] Schenk, T; Strahm, B; Kontny, U; Hufnagel, M; Neumann-Haefelin, D; Falcone, V. Disseminated Bocavirus Infection after Stem Cell Transplant. *Emerg Infect Dis*, 2007, 13(9), 1425-7.

[78] Kesebir, D; Vazquez, M; Weibel, C; Shapiro, ED; Ferguson, D; Landry, ML; et al. Human bocavirus infection in young children in the United States: molecular epidemiological profile and clinical characteristics of a newly emerging respiratory virus. *J Infect Dis*, 2006, 194(9), 1276-82.

[79] Monteny, M; Niesters, HG; Moll, HA; Berger, MY. Human bocavirus in febrile children, The Netherlands. *Emerg Infect Dis*, 2007, 13(1), 180-2.

[80] Bonvicini, F; Gallinella, G; Gentilomi, GA; Ambretti, S; Musiani, M; Zerbini, M. Prevention of iatrogenic transmission of B19 infection: different approaches to detect, remove or inactivate virus contamination. *Clin Lab*, 2006, 52(5-6), 263-8.

[81] Brauniger, S; Peters, J; Borchers, U; Kao, M. Further studies on thermal resistance of bovine parvovirus against moist and dry heat. *Int J Hyg Environ Health*, 2000, 203(1), 71-5.

[82] Weinstock, DM; Boeckh, M; Boulad, F; Eagan, JA; Fraser, VJ; Henderson, DK; et al. Postexposure prophylaxis against varicella-zoster virus infection among recipients of hematopoietic stem cell transplant: unresolved issues. *Infect Control Hosp Epidemiol*, 2004, 25(7), 603-8.

[83] Mantadakis, E; Anagnostatou, N; Danilatou, V; Markaki, EA; Spanaki, AM; Briassoulis, G; et al. Fulminant hepatitis due to varicella zoster virus in a girl with acute lymphoblastic leukemia in remission: report of a case and review. *J Pediatr Hematol Oncol*, 2005, 27(10), 551-3.

[84] Ishida, Y; Tauchi, H; Higaki, A; Yokota-Outou, Y; Kida, K. Postexposure prophylaxis of varicella in children with leukemia by oral acyclovir. *Pediatrics*, 1996, 97(1), 150-1.

[85] Rowland, P; Wald, ER; Mirro, JR; Jr.; Yunis, E; Albo, VC; Wollman, MR; et al. Progressive varicella presenting with pain and minimal skin involvement in children with acute lymphoblastic leukemia. *J Clin Oncol*, 1995, 13(7), 1697-703.

[86] Hill, G; Chauvenet, AR; Lovato, J; McLean, TW. Recent steroid therapy increases severity of varicella infections in children with acute lymphoblastic leukemia. *Pediatrics*, 2005, 116(4), e525-9.

[87] Mendelson, GM; Roth, CE; Wreghitt, TG; Brown, NM; Ziegler, E; Lever, AM. Nosocomial transmission of measles to healthcare workers. Time for a national screening and immunization policy for NHS staff? *J Hosp Infect*, 2000, 44(2), 154-5.

[88] Rivera, ME; Mason, WH; Ross, LA; Wright, HT; Jr. Nosocomial measles infection in a pediatric hospital during a community-wide epidemic. *J Pediatr*, 1991, 119(2), 183-6.

[89] Tennenberg, AM; Brassard, JE; Van Lieu, J; Drusin, LM. Varicella vaccination for healthcare workers at a university hospital: an analysis of costs and benefits. *Infect Control Hosp Epidemiol*, 1997, 18(6), 405-11.

[90] Weber, DJ; Rutala, WA; Hamilton, H. Prevention and control of varicella-zoster infections in healthcare facilities. *Infect Control Hosp Epidemiol*, 1996, 17(10), 694-705.

[91] American, Academy of Pediatrics. Infection prevention and control in pediatric ambulatory settings. *Pediatrics*, 2007, 120(3), 650-65.

[92] Bryant, KA; Stover, B; Cain, L; Levine, GL; Siegel, J; Jarvis, WR. Improving influenza immunization rates among healthcare workers caring for high-risk pediatric patients. *Infect Control Hosp Epidemiol*, 2004, 25(11), 912-7.

[93] Hoffmann, CJ; Perl, TM. The next battleground for patient safety: influenza immunization of healthcare workers. *Infect Control Hosp Epidemiol*, 2005, 26(11), 850-1.

[94] Simeonsson, K; Summers-Bean, C; Connolly, A. Influenza vaccination of healthcare workers: institutional strategies for improving rates. *N C Med J*, 2004, 65(6), 323-9.

[95] LaRussa, P; Steinberg, S; Meurice, F; Gershon, A. Transmission of vaccine strain varicella-zoster virus from a healthy adult with vaccine-associated rash to susceptible household contacts. *J Infect Dis*, 1997, 176(4), 1072-5.

[96] Tablan, OC; Anderson, LJ; Besser, R; Bridges, C; Hajjeh, R. Guidelines for preventing health-care-associated pneumonia, 2003: recommendations of CDC and the Healthcare Infection Control Practices Advisory Committee. *MMWR Recomm Rep*, 2004, 53(RR-3), 1-36.

[97] Brankston, G; Gitterman, L; Hirji, Z; Lemieux, C; Gardam, M. Transmission of influenza A in human beings. *Lancet Infect Dis*, 2007, 7(4), 257-65.

[98] Bridges, CB; Kuehnert, MJ; Hall, CB. Transmission of influenza: implications for control in health care settings. *Clin Infect Dis*, 2003, 37(8), 1094-101.

[99] Tellier, R. Review of aerosol transmission of influenza A virus. *Emerg Infect Dis*, 2006, 12(11), 1657-62.

In: Cross Infections: Types, Causes and Prevention
Editors: Jin Dong and Xun Liang
ISBN: 978-1-60741-467-4
© 2009 Nova Science Publishers, Inc.

Chapter VI

Enterotoxigenic *Staphylococcus aureus* and Bovine Mastitis: A Public Health Problem

Maria de Lourdes Ribeiro de Souza da Cunha*
Department of Microbiology and Immunology, Biosciences Institute, São Paulo State University (UNESP), Botucatu, SP, Brazil

Abstract

Mastitis is an infectious disease that is highly prevalent in dairy herds and responsible for financial losses worldwide. Most losses are attributed to subclinical mastitis, which is only detectable with indirect diagnostic tests using milk samples. *Staphylococcus aureus* is the main causative agent of mastitis in dairy herds. The udder of infected cows is the main reservoir of *S. aureus*, which can be transmitted to other cows in the herd. There are numerous sources of *S. aureus*, including stables and feeds, equipment and animal skin of cattle and other species, as well as humans themselves. Teat skin has been implicated as an important reservoir for intramammary infection; however, transmission from man has been proposed. Various virulence factors are responsible for the symptoms and severity of infections caused by *S. aureus*. These factors include hemolysins, leukocidins and a group of toxic pyrogenic superantigens consisting of the toxic shock syndrome toxin 1 (TSST-1) and staphylococcal enterotoxins, which cause staphylococcal food intoxication. *S. aureus* enterotoxins are the most frequent cause of food intoxication, with reports of cases due to food manipulation after heat treatment. Heat destroys the vegetative bacterial microbiota in food, and non-competitive staphylococci, introduced by inadequate manipulation, may grow. Food intoxication is the result of the ingestion of foods contaminated with enterotoxigenic *S. aureus* during or after processing, inappropriate management or even inadequate refrigeration, enabling the growth of microorganisms and the production and release of toxins into the food which, when ingested, will produce all characteristic signs

* Corresponding Author: Departamento de Microbiologia e Imunologia, Instituto de Biociências, Universidade Estadual Paulista (UNESP), Botucatu, SP, Brasil. Caixa Postal 510, CEP 18618-000. Tel. 55 (14) 3811-6058 Fax:55 (14) 3815-3744. E-mail: cunhamlr@ibb.unesp.br

and symptoms. Staphylococcal enterotoxins are primarily found in foods that contain proteins and carbohydrates, such as dairy products, pastries, processed meat, mayonnaise, and salads. Inadequate manipulation of the product may increase the population of staphylococci until the time of pasteurization, implying the possibility of production of enterotoxins that are stable at high temperatures. Thus, pasteurized milk would be free of microorganisms, but not of enterotoxins. This milk may subsequently be offered to children who depend on it for their growth, a fact representing a serious public health problem. The objective of this chapter is to provide data for a better understanding of the pathogenesis and microbial properties that contribute to the persistence of *S. aureus* in dairy cattle herds.

Introduction

Bovine mastitis is the most prevalent infectious disease in dairy herds worldwide. It is characterized by inflammation in the mammary gland and generally triggered by microbial infection. Mastitis can be classified in two forms: clinical mastitis, in which clinical, local or systemic signs are observed, in addition to visual alterations in milk, which may present, lumps, pus and blood, and subclinical mastitis, which is only detectable with the use of indirect diagnostic tests applied to milk. Subclinical mastitis is much more prevalent than the clinical form, and it is characterized by alterations in milk composition, such as the increased number of somatic cells and chlorine and sodium content, in addition to decreased casein, lactose and fat content, thus leading to reduction in milk yield and quality as well as causing lower industrial production and financial loss to farmers worldwide.

The financial loss caused by bovine mastitis results from the reduction in yield and quality of milk and dairy products, in addition to the untimely disposal of animals, cost of medication and services. Public-health aspects concerning the dissemination of pathogenic microorganisms to humans by milk, or of its toxins, in addition to antibiotic residue that may be present in that type of food, must also be taken into account.

Most loss is attributed to subclinical mastitis, and *Staphylococcus aureus* is the main organism causing mastitis in dairy herds. The udder of infected cows is the major reservoir of *S. aureus*, which can be transmitted to other cows in the herd. There are numerous sources of *S. aureus*, including stables and feeds, equipment and animal skin of cattle and other species, as well as humans themselves. Teat skin has been implicated as an important reservoir for intramammary infection; however, transmission from man has been proposed.

The eradication of intrammamary infection by this agent is difficult to achieve, a fact that has been partly attained in some countries thanks to the rigorous control programs that have been established. Infections originating from external sources to the mammary gland may hinder infection control.

Staphylococcal Mastitis

S. aureus is the major microorganism causing infectious mastitis. It is the most prevalent in herds worldwide and poses the most difficulties for treatment due to its high resistance to antibiotics [1]. Coherently, *S. aureus* is also the pathogenic microorganism most frequently isolated from raw milk [2].

Data in the literature indicate a potential risk to human health in association with the consumption of milk from contaminated herds, since most of the diagnosed cases of mastitis are of the subclinical type, that is, from animals that do not show visible alterations in the mammary gland or in milk [1]. The intrammamary infections caused by *S. aureus* present important implications in public health, considering that toxins can be excreted in milk and remain stable in the products offered for consumption.

S. aureus is widely distributed in dairy herds, and the probability of contaminating raw milk with the resulting production of enterotoxins is rather high. In bovines, Kenny et al.[3] reported that at least 28.6% of the strains isolated from the udder secreted one or more toxins. Matsunaga et al. [4], however, found 34.5% of enterotoxigenic strains. In a study conducted by SÁ et al. [5] for determining the occurrence of enterotoxigenic *S. aureus* in milk samples isolated from animals with subclinical mastitis, the authors obtained 4.39% of toxigenic samples.

According to data from CDC [6], it is estimated that 185,060 intoxication cases occur in the United States every year, resulting in 1,753 hospitalizations that lead to 3 deaths. From 1993 to 1997, 42 outbreaks of staphylococcal intoxication were reported in the United States; 1,413 cases of the disease were associated, and of these, one resulted in death.

Because it is not a compulsorily reported disease in Brazil, the country shows underestimated rates of staphylococcal intoxication. Due to the low severity of the intoxication and the self-limiting character of the disease, with mild and short-lasting symptomatology, the cases and outbreaks of this intoxication type rarely cause the people involved to seek medical care, which makes hospitalization rates and the resulting report to remain relatively low. Additionally, most of the outbreaks occur in households and involve a restricted number of individuals. Reports of staphylococcal intoxication eventually take place when it involves a large number of people. According to data from the Health Surveillance Department [7], 496 outbreaks of staphylococcal intoxication occurred from 1999 to 2005 in Brazil, which was exceeded only by *Salmonella* infection. The foods frequently associated with this type of intoxication include milk and other dairy products, such as cheese, cream, and chocolate items, involved in 228 outbreaks from a total of 3,151 outbreaks of diseases transmitted by food in which the type of food implicated in the outbreaks from 1999 to 2005 was determined. Milk contamination with *S. aureus* may occur by two main routes: through the incorporation of microorganisms present in the udder, directly into the milk; or through the contact of milk with utensils and equipment contaminated during milking, collection or storage operations [1]. In the latter case, the importance of man as a reservoir for *S. aureus* and main disseminator of the microorganism in food, in a general fashion, is noteworthy [8]. Studies report that 20 to 50% of normal individuals carry this microorganism in the nasal vestibule and oropharynx [9]. The strains in the nose may pass to the hands, fingers, face and skin and eventually contaminate the air, water, soil, food and any other surface or object that may have been in contact with their carrier [8].

In São Paulo state, Brazil, 25 outbreaks of *S. aureus* intoxication, involving 200 individuals, were reported from 2001 to 2002 [10]. In the state of Minas Gerais, according to reports by Ezequiel Dias Foundation – FUNED, 12,820 people were intoxicated and 17 died after ingesting food contaminated by staphylococcal enterotoxins (SE) from 1995 to 2001 [11].

The *Staphylococcus* genus comprises various species and subspecies that are widely distributed in nature and mainly found in the skin and mucosal membranes of birds and mammals [12]. Since its proposition, in 1884, by Rosenbach, the *Staphylococcus* genus has been classified within the Micrococcaceae family. It was only in the past decade, with the advancement of molecular biology, genetic studies, profiles of fatty acids, composition of the cell wall and the studies on 16S ribosomal RNA, that the *Staphylococcus* was included in a new family: Staphylococcaceae [13]. Up to this date, 41 species have been described within the genus [14, 15], most of which are coagulase-negative, since that enzyme is exclusively synthesized by *S. aureus*, *S. schleiferi* subsps. *coagulans*, *S. intermedius, S. hyicus* and *S. delphini* [14]. Approximately half of the coagulase-negative staphylococcus (CNS) species naturally colonize humans and animals, among which are *S. epidermidis, S. haemolyticus, S. saprophyticus, S. cohnii, S. xylosus, S. capitis, S. warneri, S. hominis, S. simulans*, *S. caprae*, *S. lugdunensis* and *S. schleiferi*, *S. gallinarum* as well as others [12].

Staphylococci are Gram-positive, immovable, facultatively anaerobic cocci showing a fermentative metabolism and producing acid rather than gas. They are not photosynthetic or sporulated, but catalase-positive and capable of growing in medium containing 10% sodium chloride. They are mesophyll microorganisms with a growth temperature of 7 to 48° C, and optimal growth at 37° C; pH in the range of 4.0 to 10.0, with optimal conditions from 6.0 to 7.0 [12].

Staphylococci grow rapidly in most bacterial media. The colonies in solid media are round, smooth, raised and glistening. They produce a carotenoid pigment only when in aerobiosis, which is intensified in media containing high saline concentration. Their capacity of developing in media containing high NaCl concentration in addition to that of presenting certain tolerance to potassium tellurite and lithium chloride are useful in the preparation of selective media.

In the *Staphylococcus* genus, *Staphylococcus aureus* has always been the most important species in relation to a number of infections and intoxications in humans and animals. Various virulence factors are responsible for the symptoms and severity of infections caused by *S. aureus*. The cells of *Staphylococcus aureus* show surface components and produce various extracellular substances which contribute to their virulence. Some *S. aureus* samples have a polysaccharide capsule that provides them with greater resistance to phagocytosis than in those non-capsulated. The capsule hinders the bacterium's adherence to the phagocyte. Peptidoglycans activate the alternative route of the complement, thus causing an inflammatory reaction by the host. The teichoid acids (ribitol polymers) are components of the *S. aureus*' cell wall and act on the adherence to the host's mucosal surfaces. Protein A is found in most *S. aureus* samples, and its property is the capacity to bind to the Fc portion of IgG, thus preventing phagocytosis. Most protein A is found on the bacterial wall and covalently bound to the peptidoglycan. During *in-vitro* cellular growth, protein A is released to the culture medium, which may also occur in the inflammatory processes caused by this bacterium. Protein A acts as a virulence factor and interferes with the opsonization and ingestion of the microorganism by polymorphonuclear leukocytes. Adesins are proteins that are also anchored on the peptidoglycan and promote tissue colonization by *S. aureus*, making such organisms capable of binding to fibronectins and laminin (glycoproteins in the cellular membrane).

S. aureus produces a number of extracellular enzymes. Most of them have been reported to participate in the infections caused by this microorganism. The best-known of such enzymes is coagulase due to the fact that its presence characterizes the species. Although the suffix "ase" suggests that it hydrolyzes clots, its effect is exactly the opposite, that is, it coagulates plasma. *S. aureus* strains show two forms of coagulase: bound (also referred to as clumping factor) and free coagulase. Coagulase bound to the staphylococcal cell wall can directly convert fibrinogen into insoluble fibrin, causing staphylococci to clump. Free coagulase reacts with pro-thrombin, thus forming staphylothrombin, which, in turn, catalyzes the conversion of fibrinogen into insoluble fibrin. The role of coagulase in the pathogeny of the disease is speculative, but both free and bound coagulase can cover bacterial cells with fibrin and make them resistant to opsonization and phagocytosis.

All staphylococci produce catalase, an enzyme that catalyzes the conversion of hydrogen peroxide into water and oxygen. Catalase protects organisms from toxic hydrogen peroxide which accumulates during bacterial metabolism and within phagocytic cells, after phagocytosis.

Fibrinolysin is the enzyme that activates plasminogen, a precursor existing in plasma, and generates a proteolyctic enzyme (plasmin) which is capable of dissolving fibrin, thus helping with propagation through tissues. It is produced by almost all *S. aureus* strains.

Hyaluronidase in an enzyme that hydrolyzes hyalurinic acid, a component of the intracellular matrix of connective tissue. Hyaluronidase facilitates *S. aureus* dissemination in the tissue. More than 90% of *S. aureus* strains produce this enzyme. All *S. aureus* and more than 30% of coagulase-negative staphylococci (CNS) produce various different lipases. As indicated by their name, these enzymes hydrolyze lipids, which is essential for staphylococcal survival in the sebaceous regions of the body. It is believed that these enzymes are necessary for staphylococcal invasion into cutaneous and subcutaneous tissues and for the formation of superficial cutaneous infections (as for instance furuncles and carbuncules). Another *S. aureus* marker is the production of nucleases, of which the most important is the thermostable nuclease that hydrolyzes free DNA.

S. aureus produces various toxins that act through different mechanisms. Some are cytotoxins which affect cell membranes and form pores on them, thus promoting the exit of cellular content and leading to cell death. These factors include α, β, γ and δ hemolysins and leukocidins. They were firstly described as hemolysins based on their capacity to lyse red blood cells, but since their activity is not restricted to such cells, the term cytolytic toxin was introduced. Four hemolysins are produced by *S. aureus*: alpha (α), beta (β), delta (δ) and gamma (γ). Alpha toxin (α) has lethal action on a wide variety of cell types, including the erythrocytes of various animal species, leukocytes, platelets, fibroblasts and hepatocytes. It is believed that the alpha toxin is an important tissue-lesion mediator in the staphylococcal disease.

The beta toxin (β) is also referred to as sphingomyelinase C, a toxic thermolabile protein to various cells, including red blood cells, leukocytes and macrophages. This enzyme catalyzes the hydrolysis of phospholipids in the membrane of susceptible cells, and the lysis volume is proportional to the concentration of sphingomyelin exposed on the cell surface. The beta toxin, together with the alpha toxin, seems to be responsible for the tissue destruction and abscess formation which is characteristic of staphylococcal diseases.

The delta toxin (δ) is a large thermostable protein that possesses a wide cytolytic-activity spectrum. The toxin breaks cell membranes through a detergent-type action. The direct action of the toxin on the cell membrane alters the transport of ions, leading to increased levels of

AMPc. The delta toxin seems to play an important role in the pathogeny of intestinal diseases, which may vary from acute diarrhea to severe enteritis. The gamma toxin (γ) is capable of lysing various types of red blood cells, including human, sheep and rabbit cells.

Leukocidin, referred to as Panton-Valentine Leukocidin (PVL), has exclusive and selective action on human and rabbit neutrophils and macrophages, exerting a direct toxic effect on the cell membranes of human polymorphonuclear leukocytes and causing cytoplasmic degranulation. Leukocidin enables organisms to fight against phagocytosis and subsequent bacterial cell death. It is codified by genes *pvl*, *luk*S-PV and *luk*F-PV. *In-vivo* studies have shown that, when intradermally administered in rabbits, PVL caused severe inflammatory lesions, including capillary dilation, chemotaxia, PMN infiltrate, PMN karyorrhexis and skin and tissue necrosis. Clinically, it has been related to a severe form of necrotizing pneumonia and necrotic skin lesions, such as furuncles and carbuncules [16].

PVL toxicity requires the interaction of component S (31 to 32 kDa) with the PMN membrane receptor, followed by the binding of component F (35 kDa). It has been shown by various studies and techniques (flow cytometry, spectrofluorometry, immunologic studies) that this sequential biding of S and F proteins to the surface of the target membrane induces various cell responses, thus forming pores, which are specific for the traffic of monovalent cations [17]. The binding, oligomerization and formation of the pre-pore and the insertion into membranes are generally admitted as essential phases prior to the formation of the functional pore [18].

Enterotoxins (referred to by the acronym SE: staphylococcal enterotoxins) are the direct cause of staphylococcal food poisoning. The staphylococcal enterotoxins began to be described in 1959 by Bergdoll and collaborators, and, at present, there are 18 serologically distinct enterotoxins designated by the letters SEA, SEB , SEC, SED, SEE, SEG, SEH, SEI, SEJ, SEK, SEL, SEM, SEN, SEO, SEP, SEQ, SER, SEU [19]. SECs are a group of toxins of chromosomal origin. They are highly conserved and present three different subtypes: SEC_1, SEC_2 and SEC_3, based on the differences of antigenic determinants [20]. Other molecular varieties of EEC have been described according to the animal host to which they are related, SEC_{bovine}, SEC_{canine}, SEC_{ovine} [21]. Among the staphylococcal enterotoxins, SEA is the most commonly involved in food-intoxication outbreaks, followed by SED [8]. Additionally, *S. aureus* is capable of producing more than one enterotoxin simultaneously. The simultaneous production of different toxin types can increase their isolated toxigenic effects, thus suggesting that such co-production may play an important role in the pathogeny of intrammamary infections produced by this microorganism [1].

Staphylococcal enterotoxins (SES) are water-soluble, globular proteins with a molecular weight between 26,000 and 29,000 daltons. They are rich in lysine, aspartic and glutamic acid, and have two cysteines forming a disulphate bridge [22]. They are relatively resistant to heat and proteolytic enzymes trypsin, pepsin, renin and papain, which enables them to pass through the gastrointestinal tract without activity loss [9]. The enterotoxins are thermostable, and their inactivation depends on the temperature as well as on the purity, composition and pH of the medium [23]. Studies conducted by these authors have shown that SEC is the most thermostable of enterotoxins, followed by SEB and SEA. According to [24], three to eight minutes and a temperature of 121°C would be necessary to inactivate the toxin. According to the FDA [25], the staphylococcal toxin is sensitive at 98.9 °C for 68.5 minutes or at 126.7°C for 6.2 minutes.

Although staphylococcal enterotoxins are similar to one another in structure and biological properties [20], they differ in relation to genetic location, their production and gene-regulation mechanism. Many of the genes responsible for the virulence factors are located in genetic elements that are strain-specific. Genetic elements such as plasmids, transposons, bacteriophages and, more recently, pathogenicity islets have been described for *S. aureus* [26].

The genes responsible for the production of enterotoxins have been described since 1984, when it was possible to clone SEA by transferring chromosomal DNA from an enterotoxigenic *S. aureus* to an *Escherichia coli* strain [27]. Genes *sea* and *see*, responsible for SEA and SEE production, respectively, are carried in prophages [28]. Genes *sed* and *sej*, determinants of toxins SED and SEJ, are of plasmidial origin. Gene *seb*, responsible for SEB production may be of chromosomal origin [29] or may be carried by plasmids [30] or transposons. Genes *sec-1* and *sed* are carried by plasmids. Table 2 shows the percent identity of the amino acid sequence (aas) of different staphylococcal enterotoxins. SEA shows 83% homology with SEA; SEB presents 68% homology with SEC-1. SEJ shows similar sequences to those of SEA, SEE and SED, corresponding to 64, 63 and 51%, respectively. PCR amplification suggests that gene *sej* may be present in all plasmids that codify SED [31, 32].

Toxin 1 of the Toxic Shock Syndrome (TSST-1) and staphylococcal enterotoxins (SEs), which cause staphylococcal food intoxication, form the group of superantigens [14]. Enterotoxins and TSST-1, being superantigens, directly bind to the class-II molecule of the main histocompatibility complex (MHC II), without the typical processing of normal antigens, resulting in the stimulation of many T cells and, therefore, in the excessive production of cytokines, such as interleukin I (IL-1), IL-2, gamma interferon (IFN-ϒ) and the tumor necrosis factor (TNF-α) [20].

Various regulatory systems are involved in the determination of *S. aureus* virulence. Of all such existing systems, the best characterized are *agr* and *sar* [33]. The *agr* system, by interacting with *sar*, controls the transcription of an mRNA, which is referred to as RNAIII and controls the expression of *S. aureus* virulence genes. The expression of genes that codify adesins occurs in the stationary phase of bacterial growth whereas the RNAIII molecule inhibits the expression of genes codifying adesins and induces the expression of those codifying toxins. The *agr* system is controlled by *quoruom sensing*, a language used by bacteria, which, when in high cellular density, can "feel" what is the best moment to express the factors and virulence, and thus ensure that the conjoint attack to the host will be efficient.

In addition to the various systems responsible for the regulation of *Staphylococcus* spp. virulence factors, some environmental factors, such as inoculum size, oxygen concentration, temperature, pH, NaCl concentration, mineral ions and medium composition act as external stimuli in regulating the system, thus interfering in the production of the secreted proteins, regardless of *agr* or interacting with it [34].

Water activity is considered to be one of the major factors in staphylococcal enterotoxin production, and minimum activity is of 0.86 [35]. As regards pH, it is observed that enterotoxin production does not occur in pH higher than 9.0 or lower than 5.0, and it is decreased by 50% in pH 8.0 [36]. Concerning the number of staphylococcal cells necessary for enterotoxin production in sufficient amounts to cause gastroenteritis, it is considered that a number of approximately 10^6 UFC/g or ml will be necessary [37]. The capacity to produce one or more enterotoxins is found in 30 to 50% of *S. aureus* strains.

The amount of enterotoxin expressed by each enterotoxin class also differs. Bergdoll [22] described that SEB and SEC are expressed in larger amounts than other enterotoxins, frequently in the order of 100 μg/ml of culture supernatant, whereas the maximum production obtained for SEA, SED and SEE is usually less than 10 μg/ml.

The amount of enterotoxin necessary to cause intoxication has not yet been exactly established. It is considered that the ingestion of food contaminated with staphylococcal enterotoxin in concentrations of 1ng/g can lead to the onset of symptoms. This value was estimated from an outbreak occurring in the United States which was attributed to chocolate milk and whose samples showed SEA in the mean level of 144 ng/package [38]. However, factors such as age, body mass and an individual's physical conditions will influence the development of symptoms.

The main symptoms, which occur from 1 to 6 hours after toxin ingestion, are nausea, vomiting, diarrhea, abdominal pain and headache. Clinical conditions are relatively mild, lasting from a few hours to one day, and at times may be severe and require hospitalization. This occurs due to the amount ingested and the individual's susceptibility, including dehydration, cephalea, sudoresis and body temperature alteration. Deaths are rare, but have occurred to children and the elderly [39].

TSST-1 produced by *S. aureus* isolated from clinical and subclinical bovine-mastitis cases is also noteworthy. TSST-1 is responsible for the Toxic Shock Syndrome (TSS) in humans. It an acute systemic disease characterized by fever, arterial hypotension, cutaneous rashes and skin scaling. The first detection of TSST-1 produced by animal-originated *S. aureus* was reported by Jones and Wieneke [40]. More recent studies performed with *S. aureus* isolated from clinical and subclinical cases of bovine mastitis showed that 43% of the isolates produced TSST-1 [41].

At first, enterotoxin production capacity was considered to be characteristic of *S. aureus*. However, some authors have reported the isolation of other coagulase-positive enterotoxigenic species, such as *S. intermedius* and *S. hyicus* [42]. Due to this correlation, in 2001, the Brazilian Legislation of Microbiological Food Standards was altered, and the determination of *S. aureus* was replaced by the enumeration of "coagulase-positive staphylococcus" (CPS) [43]. Nevertheless, the coagulase-positive staphylococcus enumeration in food still underestimates the amount of potentially enterotoxigenic *Staphylococcus* spp.

Research on coagulase-negative staphylococci has shown toxigenic potential in laboratory culture media [44] and in food, including *S. cohnii*, *S. epidermidis*, *S. saprophyticus*, *S. sciuri*, *S. warneri*, *S. chromogenes*, *S. lentus*, *S. xylosus* and *S. lugdunensis* [44, 45, 46]. The literature also reports three staphylococcal intoxication outbreaks associated with coagulase-negative species. The first occurred in Osaka, Japan in 1959 [47] and involved 40 students who had breakfast and lunch at a hotel. Only three coprocultures were positive for growth of coagulase-nonproducing staphylococci. The enterotoxin production tests were performed by administering cultures of such staphylococci to two kittens, which vomited after 30 minutes.

The second outbreak took place in the United States in 1969 and involved 145 persons who had meals at the same restaurant. The meat consumed in the meals showed the presence of EEA-producing *S. apidermidis*. The same species was isolated from the cook's hands. Concentrated cultures of staphylococci isolated from the meat and its manipulator were administered to monkeys, which showed emesis [48].

The third outbreak occurred in Brazil in 1999 and was associated with the consumption of raw milk [11] from which it was not possible to isolate any coagulase-positive species. Only EEC- and EED-producing coagulase-negative staphylococci (CNS) were isolated in counts greater than 2.0 X 10^8 UFC/g. Milk contamination occurred due mastitis in dairy cattle. Later studies concluded that it was a case of contamination with *S. epidermidis*.

Conclusion

In view of these facts and of the possible dissemination of staphylococcal gastroenteritis, not only through the consumption of contaminated raw milk, but also of thermally treated milk and other dairy products containing thermostable enterotoxins, preventing and controlling intrammamary infections in herds is of utmost importance in order to improve the quality of products provided to the population.

Many toxins and proteins are regulated by global genes in staphylococcal infections. Such genes are referred to as *agr* and *sar*. The *agr* locus is known for activating the expression of exotoxin genes, such as alpha-hemolysin, beta-hemolysin, TSST-1 toxin and enterotoxins, and for negatively regulating the synthesis of surface proteins, such as protein A and adesins. Various studies on these proteins and genes have been described in infections in humans; however, there are few reports on infections in animals, particularly in cows with mastitis. In order to learn about the etiologic complexity of mastitis caused by *Staphylococcus,* it is necessary to achieve the phenotypic and genotypic characterization of the lineages involved in the cases of such disease as well as of that of the milking equipment. Specific properties of the persistent strains of *S. aureus* are capable of promoting chronic infections in herds despite control methods. The knowledge on the *S. aureus* distribution in dairy herds can contribute to the formulation of strategies to reduce infection dissemination in properties. The knowledge on the molecular profile of *Staphylococcus aureus* clones allows for epidemiological studies on the dispersion of such pathogen in rural properties, with the purpose to understand the pathogeny and microbial properties that may contribute to such persistence in dairy bovine herds. Hence, strategies and protocols for mastitis prevention and control can be better designed.

Acknowledgments

Fundação de Amparo a Pesquisa do Estado de São Paulo (FAPESP).

References

[1] Fagundes, H; Oliveira, CAF. Infecções intramamárias causadas por *Staphylococcus aureus* e suas implicações em saúde pública. *Ciênc Rural,* 2004, 34, 1315-20.

[2] Zecconi, A; Hahn, G. *Staphylococcus aureus* in raw milk and human health risk. *Bull IDF,* 2000, 345, 15-8.

[3] Kenny K; Reiser RF; Bastida-Corcuera FD; Norcross N L. Production of enterotoxins and toxic shock syndrome toxin by bovine mammary isolates of *Staphylococcus aureus*. *J Clin Microbiol,* 1993. 31, 796-7.

[4] Matsunaga, T; Kamata, S; Kakiichi, N; Uchida, K. Characteristics of *Staphylococcus aureus* isolated from peracute, acute and chronic bovine mastitis. *J Vet Med Sci.* 1993, 55, 297-300.

[5] Sá, MEP; Cunha, MLRS; Elias, AO; Victória, C; Langoni, H. Importância do *Staphylococcus aureus* nas mastites subclínicas: pesquisa de enterotoxinas e toxina do choque tóxico, e a relação com a contagem de células somáticas. *Braz J Vet Res Anim Sci.* 2004, 41, 320-6.

[6] CDC. 2000. CDC surveillance summaries, March 17, 2000. *Morb. Mortal. Weekly Rep.* 49 (No. SS-1).

[7] Ministério da Saúde. Situação epidemiológica das doenças transmitidas por alimento. *Boletim Epidemiológico da Secretaria de Vigilância em Saúde* (SVS). 2005.

[8] Jay, JM. Gastrenterite estafilocócica. In: Jay, JM, editor. *Microbiologia de Alimentos.* 6ª ed., Porto Alegre: Artmed; 2005; p. 471-89.

[9] Huy, YH. Foodborne disease handbook - diseases caused by bacteria. New York: Marcel Dekker; 1994.

[10] CVE. Centro de Vigilância Epidemiológica. Secretaria do Estado de São Paulo. São Paulo, 2003.

[11] Carmo, LS. Intoxicação alimentar. Revista Minas faz Ciências. 2002, n. 11, p. 1-2, jun./ago, 2002.

[12] Kloos, WE; Bannerman, TL. *Staphylococcus* and *Micrococcus.* In: Murray PR; Baron EJ; Pfaller MA; Tenover FC; Yolken RH; Editors. *Manual of clinical microbiology.* Washington: American Society for Microbiology; 1999; p. 264-82.

[13] Garrity GM; Holt JG. The road map to the manual. In: Boone, DR; Castenholz, RW; Editors. *Bergey's Manual of Systematic Bacteriology,* New York: Berlim: Springer-Verlag, 2001, 1, 119-66.

[14] Bannerman, TL. *Staphylococcus*, *Micrococcus*, and other catalase-positive cocci that grow aerobically. In: Murray PR, Baron EJ, Jorgensen JH, Pfaller MA, Yolken RH, Editors. *Manual of clinical microbiology.* Washington: American Society for Microbiology, 2003, p. 384-404.

[15] Euzéby (JP.): List of Bacterial Names with Standing in Nomenclature: a folder available on the Internet. *Int. J. Syst. Bacteriol.*, 1997, 47, 590-592. (List of Prokaryotic Names with Standing in Nomenclature. Last full update November 05, 2008. URL: http://www.bacterio.net)

[16] Bocchin, CE; Hulten, KG; Mason, EO; Gonzalez, BE; Hammerman, WA; Kaplan, SL. Panton-valentine leukocidin genes are associated with enhanced inflammatory response and local disease in acute hematogenous *Staphylococcus aureus* osteomyelitis in children. *Pediatrics.* 2006, 117, 433- 40.

[17] Pédelacq, JD; Maveyraud, L; Prévost, G; Baba-Moussa, L; González, A; Courcelle, E; Shepard, W; Monteil, H; Samama, JP; Mourey, L. The structure of a *Staphylococcus aureus* leucocidin component (LukF-PV) reveals the fold of the water-soluble species of a family of transmembrane pore-forming toxins. *Structure.* 1999, 7, 277-87.

[18] Baba-Moussa, L; Werner, S; Colin, DA; Mourey, L; Pédelacq, JD; Samama, JP, Sanni, A; Monteil, H; Prévost, G. Discoupling the Ca^{2+}-activation from the pore-forming function of the bi-component Panton-Valentine leucocidin in human PMNs. *FEBS Letter* .1999, 461, 280-86.

[19] Jorgensen, HJ; Mørk, T; Caugant, DA; Kearns, A; Rørvik, LM. Genetic variation among *Staphylococcus aureus* strains from Norwegian Bulk Milk. *Appl Environl Microbiol*. 2005, 71, 8352- 61.

[20] Marrack, P; Kappler, J. The staphylococcal enterotoxins and their relatives. *Science*. 1990, 248, 705-11.

[21] Marr, JC; Lyon, JD; Roberson, JR; Lupher, M; Davis, WC; Bohach, GA. Characterization of Novel Type C Staphylococcal Enterotoxins: Biological and Evolutionary Implications. *Infect Immun*. 1993, 61, 4254-62.

[22] Bergdoll, MS. *Staphylococcus aureus*. In: Doyle, M.P, editor. *Foodborne bacterial pathogens*. New York: M. Dekker, 1989, p.463-523.

[23] Notermans, S; Heuvelman, KJ; Wernsrds, K. Synthetic enterotoxin B DNA probes for detection of enterotoxigenic *Staphylococcus aureus* stranis. *Appl Environ Microbiol*. 1988, 54 , 531-3.

[24] Baird-Parker, AC. The staphylococci - an introduction. *J Appl Bacteriol*. 1990, Supplement 69, 1S-8S.

[25] FDA. Food and Drug Administration. Center for Food Safety and Applied Nutrition. *Bacterial Pathogens Growth and Inativation*. 3. ed, junho, 2001. Available at: <http:/www.seafoods.ucdavis.edu/HACCP/compendium/chapt19.htm.

[26] Macmicking, JD. Altered responses to bacterial infection and endotoxic shock in mice lacking inducible nitric oxide synthase. *Cell*. 1995, 81, 641-50.

[27] Betley, MJ; Lofdahl, S; Kreiswirth, BN; Bergdoll, MS; Novick, RP. Staphylococcal enterotoxin A gene is associated with a variable genetic element. *Proc Natl Acad Sci*. 1984, 81, 5179-83.

[28] Schad, EM; Papageorgiou, AC; Svensson, LA; Acharya, KR. A structural and functional comparison of staphylococcal enterotoxins A and C2 reveals remarkable similarity and dissimilarity. *J Mol Biol*.1997, 269, 270-80.

[29] Shafer, WM; Iandolo, JJ. Chromosomal locus for staphylococcal enterotoxin B. *Infect Immun*., 1978, 20, 73-278.

[30] Shalita, Z; Hertman, I; Sand, S. Isolation and characterization of a plasmid involved with enterotoxin B production in *Staphylococcus aureus*. *J Bacteriol*.1977, 129, 317-25.

[31] Balaban, N; Rasooly, A. Staphylococcal enterotoxins. *Int J food Microbiol*. 2000, 61, 1-10.

[32] Bennett, RW; Notermans, S; Tatini, SR. Staphylococcal enterotoxins. In: Vanderzant C, Splittstoessa, DF; editors. *Compendium of methods for the microbiological examination of foods*. Washington (DC): American Public Health Association; 1999. p.551-92.

[33] Garvis, S; Mei, JM; Ruiz-Albert, J; Holden, DW. *Staphylococcus aureus svrA*: a gene required for virulence and expression of the *agr* locus. *Microbiology*. 2002, 148, 3235-43.

[34] Chan, PF; Foster, SJ. The role of environmental factors en the regulation of virulence-determinant expression in *Staphylococcus aureus* 8325-4. *Microbiology*. 1998, 144: 2469-79.

[35] Smith, JL; Buchanan, RL; Palumbo, SA. Effect of food environmental on staphylococcal enterotoxin synthesis: a review. *J Food Prot.*1983, 46, 545-55.

[36] Troller, JA. Staphylococcal growth and productions factors control. *J Milk Food Microbiol.*1975, 37, 499-503.

[37] Bennett, RW; Monday, SR. *Staphylococcus aureus*. In: Milliotis MD; Bier JW; editors. *International Handbook of Foodborne Pathogens*. New York : Marcel Dekker, Inc., 2003, cap.4, p.41-59.

[38] Evenson, ML; Hinds, MW; Bernstein, RS; Bergdoll, MS. Estimation of human dose of staphylococcal enterotoxin A from a large outbreak of staphylococcal food poisoning involving chocolate milk. *Int J Food Microbiol.* 1988, 7, 311-6.

[39] Bennett, RW; Notermans, S; Tatini, SR. *Staphylococcal enterotoxins*. In:Vanderzant C; Splittstoessa, DF; editors. *Compendium of methods for the microbiological examination of foods*.Washington (DC): American Public Health Association; 1999. p.551-92

[40] Jones, TO; Wieneke, A.A. Staphylococcal toxic shock syndrome. *Vet Rec.* 1986, 119 , 435-6.

[41] Cardoso, HFT; Carmo, LS; Silva, N. Detecção da toxina-1 da síndrome do choque tóxico em amostras de *Staphylococcus aureus* isoladas de mastite bovina. *Arq. Bras. Med. Vet. Zootec.* 2000, 52, 7-10.

[42] Hirooka, EY; Muller, EE; Freitas, JC; Vicente, E; Yoshimoto, Y; Bergdoll MSl. Enterotoxigenicity of *Staphylococcus intermedius* of canine origin. *Int J Food Microbiol.* 1988, 7, 185-91.

[43] Brasil, Agência Nacional de Vigilância Sanitária – ANVISA, Resolução RDC n. 12, de 2 de janeiro de 2001, dispõe sobre o Regulamento Técnico sobre Padrões Microbiológicos para Alimentos, revogando a portaria SVS/MS 451, de 19 de setembro de 1997, publicado no DOU de 2 de julho de 1998. *Diário Oficial* (da União), Brasília 2 de janeiro de 2001. Dispponível em: http://www.anvisa.gov.br/legis/resol/12_01-rdc,htm. Acesso em: 6 ago.2001.

[44] Udo, EE. Enterotoxin production by coagulase-negative staphylococci in restaurant workers from Kuawait City may be a potential cause of food poisoning. *J Med Microbiol.* 1999, 48, 819-23, 1999.

[45] Vernozy, RC; Mazuy, C; Prevost, G. Lapeyre, G; Bes, C; Brun, M; Fleurette, Y; J. Enterotoxin production by coagulase-negative staphylococci isolated from goats milk and chees. *Int J Food Microbiol.* 1996, 30, 271-80.

[46] Cunha MLRS; Peresi, E; Calsolari, RAO; Araújo Jr JP. Detection of enterotoxins genes in coagulase-negative staphylococci isolated from foods. *Braz J Microbiol.* 2006, 37, 64- 69.

[47] Omori, G; Kato, YA. staphylococcal food-poisoning caused by a coagulase negative strain. *Biken's Journal.* 1959, 2, 92-6.

[48] Breckinridge, JC; Bergdoll, MS. Outbreak of food-borne gastroenteritis due to a coagulase-negative enterotoxin-producing *Staphylococcus*. *New Engl J Med.* 1971, 284, 541-3.

In: Cross Infections: Types, Causes and Prevention
Editors: Jin Dong and Xun Liang

ISBN: 978-1-60741-467-4
© 2009 Nova Science Publishers, Inc.

Chapter VII

Multi-Drug Resistant Bacteria in Severe Acute Exacerbations of Chronic Obstructive Pulmonary Disease Requiring Mechanical Ventilation: Treatment and Outcomes

Elpis Giantsou
Adult Intensive Care Unit, John Radcliffe Hospital,
Headley Way, Oxford OX3 9DU, England

Abstract

Severe acute exacerbations of chronic obstructive pulmonary disease requiring mechanical ventilation are frequently attributed to bacteria. Multi-drug resistant pathogens are common in patients with severe acute exacerbations of chronic obstructive pulmonary disease, especially when they were previously intubated or had used antibiotics. These pathogens are also associated with increased rate of initially inappropriate antibiotic therapy. Although multi-drug resistant bacteria are not independently associated with increased intensive care unit mortality, an initially inappropriate antibiotic treatment is an independent factor for intensive care unit mortality in patients with severe acute exacerbations of chronic obstructive epulmonary disease. This may be explained by the higher ventilator-associated pneumonia rates observed in these patients Ventilator-associated pneumonia is independently associated with increased intensive care unit mortality in patients with severe acute exacerbations of chronic obstructive pulmonary disease. Therefore, for mechanically ventilated patients with severe acute exacerbations of chronic obstructive pulmonary disease an initially appropriate antibiotic regimen might have beneficial impact on clinical outcomes. Given the growing antimicrobial resistance for *Streptococcus pneumoniae* and the high incidence of β-lactamase producing strains, penicillin's and macrolides may not be appropriate, whereas *Pseudomonas aeruginosa* and *Stenotrophomonas* species and therefor broad spectrum antibiotics should probably be considered. However, although an initially broad spectrum antibiotic regimen might be reasonable, there is limited evidence to support that it would improve outcomes. Therefore, the data available advise that an initially appropriate empiric antimicrobial regimen should largely rely on local microbiology and routine microbial investigations, to control for unexpected or resistant pathogens. This approach may increase the rates of an initially appropriate antimicrobial regimen, until solid evidence become available regarding the potential role of broad spectrum empiric antibiotics in severe acute exacerbations of chronic obstructive pulmonary disease requiring mechanical ventilation

Introduction

Multi-drug resistant bacterial pathogens are common in patients with severe acute exacerbations of chronic obstructive pulmonary disease (COPD) Previous use of antibiotics and endotracheal intubation are independent risk factors for multi-drug resistant bacteria on Intensive Care Unit admission. Inappropriate antibiotic therapy is significantly more frequent in patients with multi-drug resistant bacteria and independently associated with increased Intensive Care Unit mortality. This is so because, for patients with severe acute exacerbations of COPD, the administration of an initially inappropriate antibiotic therapy is associated with increased rates of ventilator-associated pneumonia, which for these patients is an independent risk factor for increased mortality rates. Given the increased frequency of multi-drug resistant bacteria an initially broad spectrum antibiotic regimen could probably be justified for patients with severe acute exacerbations of chronic obstructive pulmonary disease. However, although it is reasonable, the evidence for benefits in outcome from broad spectrum antibiotics in patients with severe acute exacerbations of COPD is far from being solid. Therefore, we need more outcome based studies to answer the question whether broad spectrum antibiotic treatment is cost effective in severe acute exacerbations of COPD. Until these studies become available the choice of antimicrobial therapy should be guided by constant study of local microbiology and individual risk factors for multi-drug resistant bacteria.

The Role of Bacteria in COPD Exacerbations

Acute exacerbations are a frequent complication of COPD [1]. An exacerbation of COPD is defined as "an event in the natural course of the disease characterized by a change in the patient's baseline dyspnea, cough and/or sputum and beyond normal day-to-day variations, which are acute in onset and may warrant a change in regular medication" [2, 3]. Severe acute exacerbations are defined as exacerbations associated with respiratory failure and account for 10% of the critically ill patients admitted to Intensive Care [1, 4]. A considerable body of evidence suggests that exacerbations consist of acute inflammation superimposed on the chronic inflammation of COPD. This is so because several inflammatory markers measured in exhaled breath, induced or expectorated sputum, bronchoalveolar lavage, or bronchial biopsy have been found to be elevated during an acute exacerbation [5, 6, 7, 8].

Acute inflammation may be triggered in COPD by a variety of stimuli which include bacterial pathogens, viruses, particulate and non-particulate air pollutants. Bacterial infections account for at least 50% of acute exacerbations of COPD, whereas infections with viral pathogens and co-infections with viral and bacterial pathogens account for the rest [9]. Co-infection with bacterial pathogens and viruses does seem to increase the severity of exacerbations of COPD or to prolong hospitalization. Co-infections with *Chlamydia pneumoniae* and bacterial pathogens have also been reported.

The role of bacterial pathogens in acute exacerbations of COPD has been assessed using sputum cultures, serologic studies, bronchoscopic sampling of lower respiratory tract and molecular epidemiology of bacterial pathogens.

Bacterial pathogens are isolated from sputum cultures in 40-60% of acute exacerbations of COPD [10]. However, the use of sputum cultures to define the cause of acute exacerbations of COPD has several limitations. Contamination of sputum samples by upper airway secretions that may contain potential pathogens is a major concern. This limitation can be overcome, when uncontaminated lower respiratory secretions are obtained by bronchoscopy and cultures are performed quantitatively. Another limitation of sputum cultures to define the cause of acute exacerbations of COPD is that the identification of pathogens as species, in the absence of strain differentiation, does not differentiate between preexisting colonization and acquisition of a new infecting strain. This limitation can be overcome by strain differentiation using molecular typing of the pathogens recovered from sputum. However, all the studies which evaluated the role of bacteria in acute exacerbations of COPD have used a single culture of sputum at the time of presentation and standard or semi-quantitative culture techniques. No study has examined multiple sputum samples from each exacerbation or applied polymerase chain reaction for bacterial antigens to sputum samples. Therefore, it is possible that if such techniques were applied a higher proportion of acute exacerbations of COPD may have had bacterial origin.

Serologic studies to bacterial antigens have been widely used to identify whether the isolated pathogens were responsible for the infectious syndrome in acute exacerbations of COPD. However, the results of these studies are difficult to interpret. This is so because the majority of these studies compared antibodies in single sera obtained from patients with sera obtained from healthy control subjects, rather than between paired sera obtained from patients before and after the exacerbation [10]. In addition, when paired sera were used, the acute sera were obtained at the time of presentation rather than before the onset of infection. Because substantial immune response could be present at the time of presentation of the exacerbation, using acute sera as pre-infection sera could confound the results. Additionally these studies have rarely used the infecting strain as antigen and immunoassays specific for antibodies to epitopes exposed on the bacterial surface.

Bronchoscopic sampling of lower respiratory tract in acute exacerbations of COPD demonstrated significant bacterial infection of the distal airways in 50% of patients with acute exacerbation of COPD [11, 12, 13, 14]. In these data acute exacerbation of COPD was associated twice more often with distal airway infection with 10^3 or more colony forming units/ml of pathogenic bacteria and four times more often with 10^4 or more colony forming units/ml of pathogenic bacteria. These studies also demonstrated that in severe acute exacerbations of COPD 30% of bacteria were *Pseudomonas aeruginosa* and Gram negative *Enterobacteriae*. These pathogens were reported to be the predominant pathogens isolated from patients with very severe underlying COPD regardless of the severity of acute exacerbation. It is not clear whether the high frequency of multi-drug resistant bacteria in patients with severe acute exacerbations of COPD is due to antibiotic selection pressure or exposure to hospital flora from frequent exacerbations or is related to a greater degree of host immune compromise. However, the consistency of these studies supports an important pathogenic role for bacteria in a considerable proportion of exacerbations of COPD [15].

Molecular epidemiology of bacterial pathogens revealed that bacteria are implicated in a substantial proportion of acute exacerbations of COPD and suggested that acquisition of a new bacterial strain with an antigenic structure new to the host and not a periodic increase in bacterial load lead to exacerbations of COPD [9]. This may explain why sputum culture studies which have included only species and not strains identification of the bacterial pathogens isolated did not find a difference in the isolation rate of bacterial pathogens between exacerbation and stable COPD.

The New Model for Bacterial Exacerbations of COPD

The new model for bacterial exacerbations of COPD suggests that acquisition of new strains of *Haemophilus influenzae*, *Moraxella catarrhalis*, *Streptococcus pneumoniae* is the predominant initiating event for an exacerbation [9]. Bacteria can be present at significant concentrations in the airways of patients with stable COPD and a specific immune response to these bacterial strains maintains the balance and keeps stable the level of inflammation [10]. Given the strain specificity of the immune response it is evident that when a new strain is acquired then the antibodies directed against antigenically diverse strains of the same species are no longer protective [16, 17]. This is translated to increased bacterial load and increased inflammation which may lead to symptoms intense enough to diagnose an exacerbation.

The association between increased bacterial load and increased airway inflammation has only recently been highlighted, when it was recognized that sputum measurements of cells and mediators may reflect the milieu of lower airways quite accurately. This has led to studies which examined the effect of bacterial exacerbation on the airway milieu and demonstrated significantly greater neutrophilic inflammation than with non-bacterial exacerbation and higher levels of sputum interleukin-8, tumor necrosis factor-α, and neutrophil elastase during bacterial exacerbation [18, 19, 20]. The association between neutrophilic airway inflammation and presence of bacteria on sputum culture supports a bacterial cause of acute exacerbations of COPD.

Exceptions from the New Model

The mechanism of acute exacerbation of COPD following the acquisition of a new antigenically diverse microbial strain may not apply to all microbial pathogens. Indeed, several reports suggest that the acquisition of a new strain is the most likely pathogenic mechanism for acute bacterial exacerbations of COPD attributed to pathogens other than *Pseudomonas aeruginosa*. This is so because the predominant mechanism for acute exacerbations of COPD attributed to *Pseudomonas aeruginosa* is reported to be a change from the biofilm state to a free-floating planktonic state [21]. This change of state of *Pseudomonas aeruginosa* has been mainly associated with the transformation of the existing strains from type-III protein non-secreting strains to type-III protein secreting strains and less with the acquisition of new antigenically diverse strains, which are usually capable of type-III protein~~s~~ secretion [22]. Although the data regarding *Pseudomonas aeruginosa* are mainly derived from patients with cystic fibrosis, recent evidence suggests that the change of *Pseudomonas aeruginosa* from the biofilm state to a free planktonic state is associated with acute exacerbation of COPD, mainly because the bacteria of the free planktonic state are usually capable of type-III protein~~s~~ secretion.

The mechanism of transformation from type-III protein non-secreting to type-III protein secreting strains may also apply in some exacerbations of COPD caused by other gram-negative *Enterobacteriae.* However, the etiologic role of *Pseudomonas aeruginosa* and other gram-negative pathogens in the exacerbations of COPD is less clearly established compared to that of *Haemophilus influenzae, Moraxella catarrhalis* and *Streptococcus pneumoniae.* Similarly, the importance of *Mycoplasma pneumoniae* and *Chlamydia pneumoniae* in severe acute excacerbations of COPD is not clearly established [23]. This is so because the relevant studies have used cultures, PCR detection or serology. It is well established that c~~C~~ultures are very difficult for these pathogens and reach very low yield whereas PCR reliability can be questioned, since there is substantial colonization by these pathogens in COPD. Additionally, s~~S~~erology requires a highly specific serologic test combined with a fourth fold increase in titer to avoid over-diagnosis of infection based on a single titer.

Antibiotics in COPD Exacerbations

The use of antibiotics in COPD exacerbations remains open to debate. The data available so far demonstrated benefits from antibiotic therapy which consisted of, shorter course of illness and faster improvement of peak flow rates in more than 80% of patients with acute exacerbation of COPD, who received antibiotics compared to placebo [24]. Potential explanations for the trials showing modest benefits with antibiotics in acute exacerbations of COPD include the following: 1) The expected benefits from antibiotics in a mucosal infection consist of faster resolution of symptoms and prevention of complications. Most studies of antibiotics in acute exacerbations of COPD have not measured the speed of resolution of symptoms, but the success of treatment at three weeks after the onset of an exacerbation. However, the immune-inflammatory response would be expected to resolve during this time period disguising any potential effect of antibiotics. 2) Many studies have included patients with mild impairment of lung function, who were likely to have a low rate of complications, making a difference from placebo prone to type II error [25]. 3) Exacerbations are non-bacterial in 20% to 50% and therefore no benefit is expected from antibiotics, predisposing to a type II error.

A meta-analysis of nine trials demonstrated that the overall standard deviation of benefits with antibiotic therapy versus placebo for the effect measured was 0.22, but seven of the nine trials included demonstrated ~~a~~ benefit from antibiotics [26]. In addition three studies have since been conducted to examine the benefits from antibiotics in acute exacerbations of COPD [27, 28, 29]. Two of them suggested that use of antibiotics was superior to placebo and that the impact was greater with more severe underlying COPD [28, 29]. Therefore, sub-setting of patients with regard to severity of COPD, may contribute to a more realistic estimation of the potential benefits derived from the use of antibiotics in acute exacerbations of COPD. This approach suggested that for patients with severe acute exacerbations of COPD requiring mechanical ventilation benefits from use of antibiotics consisted of reduced mortality by 17.5-fold and reduced use of additional antibiotics by 28.4-fold. Therefore, for patients with severe acute exacerbations of COPD the benefits from the use of antibiotics are clearly established. However, the potential role of antibiotics for non-severe acute exacerbations of COPD needs further investigation

To assess the potential role of antibiotics in the treatment of non-severe acute exacerbations of COPD, patients were stratified on the basis of clinical symptoms at presentation. The greatest benefit with antibiotics was observed for patients with non-severe acute exacerbation of COPD who had at least two cardinal symptoms (increased dyspnea, increased sputum production and/or change in sputum colour) [30]. Many international specialty societies have recommended antimicrobial therapy in acute exacerbations of COPD when they are associated with change in sputum characteristics. This is so because the importance of sputum purulence has been increasingly recognized. Acute exacerbations of COPD with purulent sputum were more likely to have positive sputum cultures and achieved higher resolution rates when treated with antibiotics.

It has been recently suggested that procalcitonin may be of use to define which patients with acute exacerbation of COPD have a higher likelihood of bacterial infection and therefore of benefit from antibiotics [31]. Data from a single-center study suggestthat procalcitonin can be used safely to reduce antibiotics by 72% in patients with low respiratory tract infection and low likelihood of bacterial infection. However, although, in that study, antibiotics use was reduced no difference was noted in clinical success rate, antimicrobial use during the subsequent six months, or in the time period until the next exacerbation. Therefore, what we need to optimize the management of non-severe acute exacerbations of COPD are more outcome–based studies, including studies that involve end points other than bacteriologic eradication and clinical cure, such as the impact of specific antibiotic choice son the long-term emergence of antibiotic resistance.

Microbiology of Severe Acute Exacerbations of COPD

Patients with severe COPD have been reported to harbor different pathogens compared to patients with less severe disease. Indeed when patients with better lung function were compared to those with worse lung function (assessed by FEV_1) the pathogens responsible for exacerbation shifted from *Streptococcus pneumoniae* and *Haemophilus influenzae* to more complex pathogens such as the *Enterobacteriae* and *Pseudomonas* species [32]. The different pathogens that patients with severe COPD may harbor compared to patients with less severe disease may account, at least in part, for the discrepancies between reports which examined the benefits from antibiotics in acute exacerbations of COPD and re-inforce the point of view that different patients may need different therapies [33].

To increase the complexity, several reports suggest that, even when the traditional pathogens such as *pneumococci*, *Haemophilus influenzae* and *Moraxella catarrhalis* are isolated from patients with severe acute exacerbations of COPD requiring mechanical ventilation, they are frequently multi-drug resistant. Thus, *pneumococci* are frequently resistant to penicillin's and other agents, while both *Haemophilus influenzae* and *Moraxella catarrhalis* species are not infrequently associated with β-lactamase production.

Reports based on large series of patients suggest that the growth of multi-drug resistant pathogens is associated with previous use of antibiotics and endotracheal intubation [34, 35]. Previous use of antibiotics is well established as a risk factor for colonization and infection with multi-drug resistant bacteria and especially with *Pseudomonas aeruginosa.* Endotracheal intubation bypasses natural host defenses, permit leakage of bacteria and secretions around the cuff into the trachea, damage the ciliated epithelium of the trachea and reduce bacterial clearance. The lack of association between previous tracheal intubation and multi-drug resistant pathogens suggested by other reports should probably be explained, at least in part, by differences in definitions used for previous intubation [36, 37].

Antibiotic Regimens for Severe Acute Exacerbations of COPD

The increasing resistance rates for *Streptococcus pneumoniae*, the high incidence of beta-lactamase producing strains of *Haemophilus influenzae* and *Moraxella catarrhalis,* and the high frequency of significant growth of *Pseudomonas aeruginosa* and other *Enterobacteriae* may contribute to high rates of an initially inappropriate empirical antibiotic treatment administered to patients with severe acute exacerbations of COPD. This is so because the usually prescribed initial empirical antibiotic therapyconsist of penicillins and macrolides, which cannot be recommended as first choice agents for multi-resistant pathogens. However, although, for patients with severe acute exacerbations of COPD the growth of multi-resistant pathogens is not independently associated with poorer outcomes, recent data suggest that the administration of an initially inappropriate antibiotic therapy is an independent risk factor for mortality [38].

Patients with severe acute exacerbations are by definition hospitalized and mechanically ventilated in an intensive care setting and therefore exposed to procedures and therapies which are well known to alter natural host defenses. Additionally, tThe innate defense mechanisms, which maintain sterility of the tracheobronchial tree, are already compromised in the inflamed airway of COPD, allowing establishment and proliferation of microbial pathogens in the lower airways, which for patients with severe acute exacerbations are highly likely to be multi-drug resistant. Therefore, it becomes evident why an initially inappropriate antibiotic therapy within an Intensive Care setting can be the determinant factor of an unfavorable outcome for patients with severe acute exacerbation of COPD. Transfer to the intensive care unit has been well documented as an independent risk factor for increased mortality in COPD.

The highest rates of ventilator-associated pneumonia among patients with initially inappropriately treated severe acute exacerbation of COPD may well explain the association of an initially inappropriate therapy with poorer clinical outcomes. The mortality attributable to ventilator-associated pneumonia has been the subject of debate and the predominant point of view was that patients die with rather than from ventilator-associated pneumonia. However, recent data suggest that mortality rates attributable to ventilator-associated pneumonia may well be pathogen dependent [39]. This is so because increased attributable mortality rates have been reported for patients with *Pseudomonas aeruginosa* ventilator-associated pneumonia. The association of other difficult to treat pathogens such as multi-resistant *Enterobacteriae* with less favorable outcome for patients with ventilator-associated pneumonia has also been previously reported. Therefore, the high frequency of multi-drug resistant bacteria in patients with severe acute exacerbations of COPD suggests that ventilator-associated pneumonia in these patients is more likely to be attributed to these pathogens and associated with an ominous prognosis.

Different Patients with COPD May Need Different Antibiotic Therapy

The choice of antibiotics for patients with severe acute exacerbations of COPD remains a difficult task. Approaches like patient stratification for the purpose of choosing antibiotic therapy during acute exacerbations of COPD identified clinical and economical benefits from the use of third line agents (quinolone, amoxicillin-clavulanate, ciprofloxacin, or azithromycin) compared to the use of first line agents (amoxicillin, trimethoprime/ sulphamethoxazole, erythromycin, or tetracyclin) for patients with severe bronchitis plus at least four exacerbations in the preceding year. The benefits were reported to be even greater when additional risk factors were present, which included the following: >10 years duration of illness; age >56 years; and multiple medical comorbidities. Following these reports guidelines have taken the approach of stratifying patients according to the risk of treatment failure [40].

A patient stratification [Figure 1], in which patient-level relies on host and pathogen features, suggested high likelihood of treatment failures with standard antibiotic treatment regimens which did not cover pathogens like *Pseudomonas aeruginosa* or other drug-resistant bacteria [8]. According to this stratification treatment failures were also more likely when patients with COPD had more severely impaired lung function, or higher frequency of exacerbations or comorbidities (particularly ischaemic heart disease). Against the patient sub-setting approach are reports which suggest that stratified antimicrobial therapy is far from being considered the gold standard of care. They claim that even with the patient stratification approach high rates of treatment failure may occur [41]. These reports suggest that we need more outcome orientated trials to prove the benefits of the stratified antimicrobial therapy in acute exacerbations of COPD.

The main contribution of patient sub-setting for the purpose of choosing therapy is that it made clear cut the wide diversity that exist between patients with acute exacerbation of COPD. The patient stratification approach pointed out the need to prescribe antibiotic agents with different patient's profiles in mind. It also suggested that the moderate benefits attributed by previous reports to the use of antibiotics in acute exacerbations of COPD might have been even greater if different antibiotics were prescribed for different patients. However, although this approach seems reasonable there are no solid data to suggest that stratified antimicrobial therapy should be considered the standard of care. Similarly, although it seems logical that broad spectrum antibiotics can be the treatment of choice for patients with severe acute exacerbations of COPD, given the documented high incidence of multi-drug resistant bacteria in these patients, there is limited evidence to support that this approach would improve clinical outcomes. Outcome-orientated studies are clearly needed to quantify the performance of stratified antimicrobial therapy in patients with acute COPD exacerbations and of broad-spectrum antibiotic agents in severe acute exacerbations of COPD.

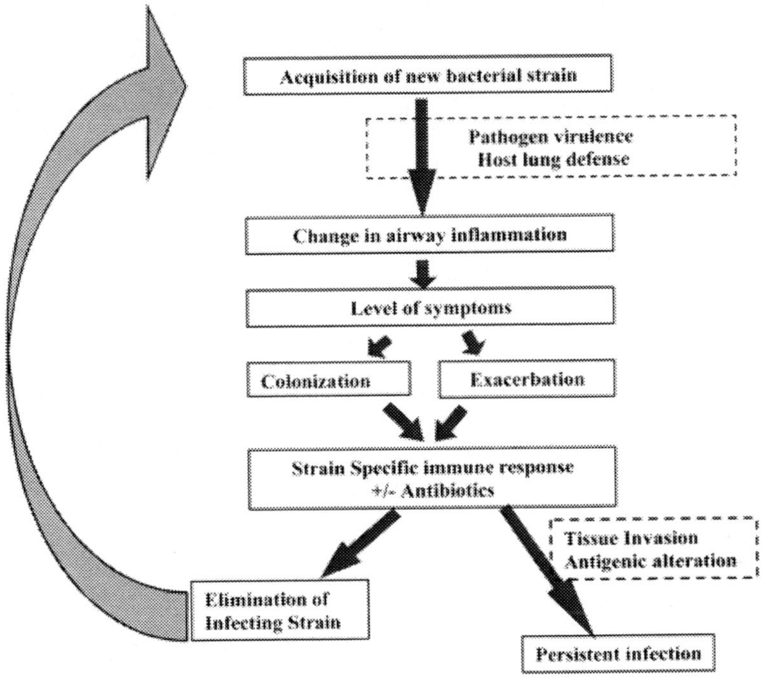

Figure 1. Proposed model of bacterial infection in chronic obstructive pulmonary disease.

Approaches to Achieve an Initially Appropriate Antibiotic Therapy

Currently available data advise that an initially appropriate antibiotic therapy may improve outcomes for patients with severe acute exacerbations of COPD. It is well established in the literature that constant study of local microbial and susceptibility patterns may help control for unexpected or resistant pathogens in the individual patient with severe acute exacerbation of COPD. The constant study of local microbiology has been charged with higher rates of an initially appropriate antibiotic therapy, which in turn have been associated with a sterilization rate of 77% [41].

Given that airway bacterial concentrations and intensity of inflammation may well be related in a stimulus-response relationship it is evident that the constant study of local microbiology through the achievement of higher rates of an initially appropriate therapy can also achieve higher eradication rates and therefore faster reduction of inflammation and resolution of COPD exacerbation. Given that exacerbations are inflammatory events it is likely that the impact of a constant study of local microbiology could be significant. It could be argued that it is not clearly established whether an intensive microbiological surveillance strategy is cost effective for patients with severe acute exacerbations of COPD, who were admitted and mechanically ventilated in an Intensive Care Unit. This is so mainly because the data on the performance of routine microbial investigations are mainly derived from patients with ventilator-associated pneumonia, some of which may had been admitted to the Intensive Care Unit for an acute exacerbation of COPD. However, the data available suggest that, until solid evidence on the performance of patients sub-setting and use of broad-spectrum antibiotic agents for severe acute exacerbations of COPD become available, the study of local microbiology and susceptibility patterns supplemented with routine microbial investigations is the best tool available. This interim policy promises to help control unexpected or resistant pathogens in the individual patient until solid data become available.

References

[1] Celi, B. R. & MacNee, W., et al. (2004). Standards for the diagnosis and treatment of patients with COPD: A summary of the ATS/ERS position paper. *Eur Respir J, 23*, 932-946.

[2] Mannino, D. M., Homa, D. M., Akinbami, L. J., Ford, E. S. & Redd, S. C. (2002). Chronic obstructive pulmonary disease surveillance-United states, 1971-2000. *MMWR Surveill Summ*, 51:1-16.

[3] Gold executive and Science Committees. Executive summary: global strategy for the diagnosis, management, and prevention of chronic obstructive pulmonary disease 2006. Available from :http://www.goldcopd.org/Guidelineitem.asp?l1=2712=1&intId=996 (accessed March 14, 2008).

[4] Esteban, A., Anzueto, A. & Frutos, A. et al (2002). Characteristics and outcomes in adult patients receiving mechanical ventilation: A 28-day international study. *JAMA, 287*, 345-355.

[5] Papi, A., Bellettato, C. M., Braccioni, F, Romagnoli, M., Casolari, P., Caramori, G., Fabbri, L. M. & Johnston, S. L. (2006). Infections and airway inflammation in chronic obstructive pulmonary disease severe exacerbations. *Am J Respir Crit Care Med, 173*, 1114-1121.

[6] Zhu, J., Qiu, Y. S, Majumdar, S., Gamble, E., Matin, D., Turato, G., Fabbri, L. M., Barnes, N., Saeta, M., Jeffery, P. K. (2001). Exacerbations of bronchitis: bronchial eosinophilia and gene expression for interleukin-4 and interleukin-5 and eosinophil chemoattractants. *Am J Respir Crit Care Med, 164*, 109-116

[7] Sethi, S., Muscarella, K., Evans, N., Klingman, K. L., Grant, B. J. B. & Murphy, T. F. (2000). Airway Inflammation and etiology of acute exacerbations of chronic bronchitis. *Chest, 118*, 1157-1565

[8] Veeramachaneni, S. B. & Sethi, S. (2006). Pathogenesis of bacterial exacerbations of COPD. COPD, *3*, 109-115.

[9] Sethi, S., Evans, N., Brydon, R. N., Grant, J. B. & Murphy, T. F. (2002). New strains of bacteria and exacerbations of Chronic Obstructive Pulmonary Disease. *N Engl J Med, 347*, 465-471.

[10] Sethi, S. & Murphy, T. S. (2001). Bacterial infections in chronic obstructive pulmonary disease in 2000: a state of the art review. *Clin Microbiol Rev, 14*, 336-363

[11] Monso, E., Ruiz, J. & Rossell, A. (1995). Bacterial infection in chronic obstructive pulmonary disease: a study of stable and exacerbated outpatients using the protected specimen brush. *Am J Respir Crit Care, 152*, 1316-1320

[12] Fagon, J. Y., Chastre, J., Trouillet, J. L., Domart, Y., Dombret, M. C, Bornet, M. & Gibert, C. (1990). Characterization of distal bronchial microflora during acute exacerbations of chronic bronchitis. *Am Rev Respir Dis, 142*, 1004-1008

[13] Soler, N., Torres, A., Ewig, S., Gonzalez, J., Celis, R., El-Ebiary, M., Hernandez, C. & Rodriguez-Roisin, R. (1998). Bronchial microbial patterns in severe exacerbations of chronic obstructive pulmonary disease duringmechanical ventilation. *Am J Respir Crit Care Med, 157*, 1498-1505

[14] Pela, R., Marchesani, F., Agostinelli, C., StaccioliD, Cesarini, L., Bassotti, C. & Sanguinetti, C. M. (1998). Airways microbial flora in COPD patients in stable clinical conditions and during exacerbations: a bronchoscopic investigation. *Monaldi Arch Chest Dis, 53*, 262-267

[15] Murphy, T. F., Sethi, S. & Niedermann, M. S. (2000). The role of bacteria in exacerbations of COPD. *Chest, 118*, 204-209.

[16] Yi, K. & SethiS Murphy, T. (1997). Humani immune response to nontypeable Haemophilus influenzae in chronic bronchitis. *I Inhnfect Dis, 176*, 1247-1252

[17] Abe, Y, Murphy, T. F., SethiS, Faden, H. S., Dmochowski, J., Harabuchi, Y. & Thanavala, Y. M. (2002). Lymphocyte proliferative response to P6 of *Haemophilus influenzae* is associated with relative protection from exacerbations of chronic obstructive pulmonary disease. *Am J Respir Crit Care Med, 165*, 957-961

[18] Sethi, S., Muscarella, K., Evans, N, Klingman, K. L, Grant, B. J. B. & Murphy, T. F. (2000). Airway inflammation and etiology of acute exacerbations of chronic bronchitis. Chest 118, 1557-1565

[19] Gompertz, S., O'Brien, C., Bayley, D. L, Hill, S. L. & Stockley, R. A. (2001). Changes in bronchial inflammation during exacerbations of chronic bronchitis. Eur Respir J 17, 1112-1119

[20] Aaron, S. D., Angel, J. B., Lunau, M., Wright, K., Fex, C., Le Saux, N. & Dales, R. E. (2001). Granulocyte inflammatory markers and airway infection during acute exacerbation of chronic obstructive pulmonary disease. *Am J Respir Crit Care Med, 163*, 349-355

[21] Song, Y., Wiener-Kronish J. P., Flanagan, J. & Lynch, S. V. (2007). Alveolar hemostasis in patients with species-specific bacterial mediated ventilator-associated pneumonia. *Crit Care Med, 35* (*2*), 652-653.

[22] Jain, M., Ramirez, D., Seshadri, R., Cullina, J. F., Powers, C. A., Sculert, G. S., Bar-Meir, M., Sullivan, C. L., McColley, S. A. & Hauser, A. R. (2004). Type III secretion phenotypes of Pseudomonas aeruginosa strains change during infection of individuals with cystic fibrosis. *J Clin Microbiol, 42*, 5229-5237.

[23] Beaty, C. D., Grayston, J. T., Wang, S. P., Kuo, C. C., Reto, C. S. & Martin, T. R. (1991). Chlamydia pneumoniae strain TWAR, infection in patients with chronic obstructive pulmonary disease. Am Rev Respir Dis 144, 1408-1410.

[24] Anthonisen, N. L., Manfreda, J., Warren, C. P. W., Hershfield, E. S, Harding, G. K. M. & Nelson, N. A (1987). Antibiotic therapy in chronic obstructive pulmonary disease. *Ann Intern Med, 106*, 196-204

[25] Kanner, R., Anthonisen, N. R. & Connett, J. E. (2001).Lower respiratory tract illnesses promote FEV_1 decline in current smokers but not ex-smokers with mild chronic obstructive pulmonary disease: results from the the lung health study. *Am J Respir Crit Care Med*, *164*, 358-364

[26] Saint, S., Bent, S., Vittinghoff, E. & Grady, D. (1995). Antibiotics in chronic obstructive pulmonary disease exacerbations: a meta analysis. *JAMA*, *273*, 957-996

[27] Sachs, A. P. E., Koeter, G. H., Groenier, K. H., van der Waaij, D., Schiphuis, J. & Jong, B. M. (1995) . Changes in symptoms , peak expiratory flow, and sputum flora during treatment with antibiotics of exacerbations with chronic obstructive pulmonary disease in general practice. Thorax 50:758-763 Nouira S, Marghli S, Belghith M, Besbes L, Elatrous S, *Abroug F*, (2001)

[28] Once daily oral ofloxacin in chronic obstructive pulmonary disease exacerbation requiring mechanical ventilation: a randomized placebo-controlled trial. *Lancet*, *358*, 2020-2025

[29] Allegra, L., Blasi, F., de Bernardi, B., Cosentini, R. & Tarsia, P. (2001). Antibiotic treatment and baseline severity of disease in acute exacerbations of chronic bronchitis: a re-evaluation of previously published data of a placebo-controlled randomized study. Pulm Pharmacol Ther 14, 149-155

[30] Stockley, R. A., O'Brien, C., Pye, A. & Hill, S. L. (2000). Relationship of sputum colour to nature and outpatient management of acute exacerbations of COPD. *Chest*, *117*, 1638-1645

[31] Stollz, D., Chris-Crain, M., Bingisser, R., Leuppi, J., Miedinger, D., Muller, C., Huber P., Muller, B. & Tamn, M. (2007). Antibiotic treatment of exacerbations of COPD: a randomized, controlled trial comparing procalcitonin-guidance with standard therapy. *Chest*, *131*, 9-19

[32] Miravitles, M., Espinosa, C., Fernandez-Laso, E., Martos, J. A., Maldonado, J. A. & Gallego, M. (1999).Relationship between bacterial flora in sputum and functional impairment in patients with severe acute exacerbations of COPD. *Chest*, *116*, 40-46

[33] Murphy, T. F. & SethiS Niederman, M. S. (2000). The role of bacteria in exacerbations of COPD. *Chest*, *118*, 204-209

[34] Nseir, S., Di Pompeo, C., Soubrier, S., Delour, P., Lenci, H., Roussel-Delvallez, M., Onimus, T., Saulnier, F., Mathieu, D. & Durocher, A. (2005). First generation fluoroquinolone use and subsequent emergence of multiple-drug resistant bacteria in the intensive care unit. *Crit Care Med*, *33*, 283-289

[35] Ewig, S., Soler N., Gonzalez, J., Celis, R., El-Ebiary, M. & Torres, A. (2000).Evaluation of antimicrobial treatment in patients with severe chronic obstructive pulmonary disease. *Crit Care Med*, *28*, 692-697

[36] Nevins M. L. & Epstein S. K. (2001). Predictors of outcome for patients with COPD requiring invasive mechanical *ventilation. Chest*, *119*, 1840–1849

[37] Shachor, Y., Liberman, D. & Tamir, A. (1989). Long-term survival of patients with chronic obstructive pulmonary disease following mechanical ventilation. *Isr J Med Sci*, *25*, 617–619

[38] Nseir, S, Di Pompeo, C, Cavestri, B, Jozefowicz, E, Nyunga, M, Soubrier, S, Roussel-Delvallez, M., Saulnier, F., Mathieu, D. & Durocher, A. (2006). Multiple-drug-resistant bacteria in patients with severe acute exacerbation of chronic obstructive pulmonary disease: Prevalence, risk factors and outcome. *Crit Care Med*, *34* (*12*), 2959-2966

[39] Combes, A, Luyt, C. E., Fagon, J. Y., Wolff, M., Trouillet, J. L. & Chastre, J. (2007). Early predictors for infetion recurrence and death in patients with ventilator-associated pneumonia. *Crit Care Med*, *35* (1). 146-154

[40] Martinez, F. J, Han, M. K., Flaherty, K. & Curtis, J. (2006). Role of infection and antimicrobial therapy in acute exacerbations of chronic obstructive pulmonary disease. *Expert Rev Anti Infect Ther*, *4*, 101-124

[41] Martinez, F. J., Grossman, R. F., Zadeikis, N, Fisher, A. C., Walker, K., Ambruzs, M. E. & Tennenberg, A. M. (2005). Patient stratification in the management of acute bacterial exacerbation of chronic bronchitis: the role of levofloxacin 750mg. *Eur Respir J*, *25*, 1001-1010

In: Cross Infections: Types, Causes and Prevention
Editors: Jin Dong and Xun Liang

ISBN: 978-1-60741-467-4
© 2009 Nova Science Publishers, Inc.

Chapter VIII

Assessment of Patient-To-Patient Transmission of Healthcare-Associated Infections: Integrating Laboratory Data with Patient-Based Surveillance

Antonella Agodi and Martina Barchitta
Department of Biomedical Sciences, University of Catania, Italy

Abstract

Epidemiological surveillance is an essential element of any infection control programme, especially in intensive care units (ICUs), to increase awareness and to identify areas for improvement. The majority of healthcare-associated infections (HAI) is of endogenous origin and therefore difficult to prevent. In contrast, exogenous infections are more likely to be preventable by standard or specific precautions devised to reduce the overall rates of nosocomial transmission. To demonstrate the exogenous route of infection, the use of highly discriminatory typing techniques is necessary: undistinguishable strains isolated from different patients may indicate that cross-transmission from one patient to another has occurred. Different methodological approaches can be used to estimate the preventable proportion of HAI. Most of the studies are laboratory driven and did not include a daily follow-up of patient status. Ideally, integrating laboratory data with active surveillance, would provide systematic observations and measurement of infection events, as well as clonality data [Scheckler et al., 1998; Agodi and Pasquarella, 2000; Agodi A, 2000]. One such approach consists in the assessment of the preventable proportion of infections integrating clonality assessment with a unit-based surveillance protocol intended for continuous surveillance, in which denominator data (patient-days) are collected for the entire unit. Although indicators generated by such a 'first-level' surveillance are not suitable for ICU benchmarking of quality of care in terms of infection control, they are appropriate for the follow-up of infections within the same unit and for regional, national and international investigation of trends for pathogen-specific infection rates. This approach has been used in a study conducted with the main aim to investigate the epidemiological impact of *Acinetobacter baumannii* HAI in a Sicilian ICU and to estimate the preventable proportion of *Acinetobacter* infections, i.e., those resulting from cross-transmission [Agodi et al., 2006].

An alternative comprehensive approach integrating the patient-based surveillance data, intended for advanced risk-adjusted comparison of infection rates between ICUs, with molecular typing data has been adopted in a recent study in order to investigate the clonality patterns sustaining the endemic *versus* the epidemic mode of transmission for acquisition of the three emerging multiresistant pathogens, *Pseudomonas aeruginosa*, *A. baumannii* and *Stenotrophomonas maltophilia*.

The present survey provides a framework for further investigation of the role of alert pathogens and/or high-risk clones together with patients' risk factor profiles for appropriate design of effective control strategies especially addressed to ICU patients.

Introduction

Epidemiological surveillance is an essential element of any infection control programme, especially in intensive care units (ICUs), to increase awareness and to identify areas for improvement. The majority of healthcare-associated infections (HAIs) is of endogenous origin and therefore difficult to prevent. In contrast, exogenous infections are more likely to be preventable by standard or specific precautions devised to reduce the overall rates of nosocomial transmission. To demonstrate the exogenous route of infection, the use of highly discriminatory typing techniques is necessary: undistinguishable strains isolated from different patients may indicate that cross-transmission from one patient to another has occurred [Weist et al., 2002]. Different methodological approaches can be used to estimate the preventable proportion of HAI. Most of the studies are laboratory driven and did not include a daily follow-up of patient status. Ideally, integrating laboratory data with active surveillance, would provide systematic observations and measurements of infection events, as well as clonality data, leading to the construction of appropriate indicators [Agodi and Pasquarella, 2000; Agodi A, 2000].

Among the most frequent pathogens isolated from ICU patients, *Pseudomonas aeruginosa* has held a nearly unchanged position during the last decades [Sehulster et al., 2004]. *Acinetobacter baumannii* has emerged globally as an increasingly important nosocomial pathogen in intensive care and burns units, and is usually resistant to most available antibiotics [Koeleman et al., 2001]. Although *Stenotrophomonas maltophilia* has been considered in the past as an unusual opportunistic pathogen with limited invasiveness, its overall isolation rate has increased and infections with *S. maltophilia* are at present difficult to manage since clinical isolates are intrinsically resistant to many broad-spectrum antibiotics [Weist et al., 2002; Zarrilli et al., 2004; Herruzo et al., 2004].

Molecular typing is an important tool to follow transmission routes of microbial pathogens that can be used in clinical settings to discriminate ongoing epidemics of an infectious agent when increased rates are observed [Renders et al., 1996; Kayabas et al., 2008]. Pulsed-field gel electrophoresis (PFGE) is the current "gold standard" for bacterial molecular typing. PFGE has been widely used for clonal analysis of *P. aeruginosa* isolates either in a specific setting or in population-based research [Kayabas et al., 2008].

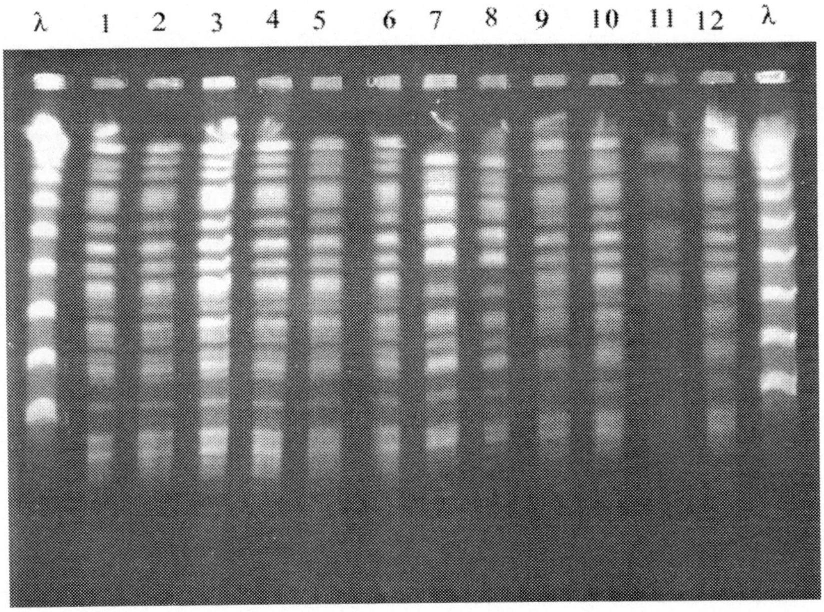

Figure 1. PFGE profiles of the outbreak strains of *P. aeruginosa*. λ ladder DNA marker; line 1. strain isolated from washing bowl; lines 2 to 12 patients' isolates.

A Survey of Studies on Cross-Transmission of HAIs

During 2001, surgery-associated *P. aeruginosa* infections increased in the heart surgery ward of the Azienda Ospedaliera Vittorio Emanuele-Ferrarotto-S.Bambino in Catania (Southern Italy). Since an outbreak was suspected, an epidemiological investigation was performed in order to trace the source of infections, identify potential reservoirs, investigate the clonal relationships among strains, and reveal the effectiveness of PFGE-based clonality definition on taking effective control measures to terminate the outbreak.

Surveillance cultures were taken from patients, health care personnel and the environment (air, surfaces and equipment). A total of 18 *P. aeruginosa* isolates were identified from 9 patients. Besides, *P. aeruginosa* was isolated from two washing bowls

The specific epidemic curve was plotted to give a visual representation of the trend of infection events over the time period. Particularly, the epidemic curve was used to provide information on the outbreak pattern of spread, magnitude and time trend. The curve showed the occurrence of an outbreak and the shape of the curve suggested a propagated or progressive source mode of epidemic transmission, reflective of the number of cases caused by person-to-person contact. Macrorestriction analysis of the *P. aeruginosa* isolates led to the identification of an unique PFGE-type responsible for the epidemic spread of *P. aeruginosa* (Figure 1).

As soon as the outbreak was identified, a multimodal infection control program was introduced in order to control the acquisition and spread of *P. aeruginosa* in the ward, including review of all healthcare procedures, training of staff in the correct washing of hands, introduction of alcohol-based antiseptic gel, enhanced cleaning and disinfection of medical equipment and ward and use of single-patient medical instruments and washing bowls. In the months following the implementation of the above described measures, a decrease in the incidence of recovery of new *P. aeruginosa* isolates was observed. In conclusion, a nosocomial outbreak should be identified immediately, and infection control measures should be carried out adequately. Molecular typing methods can help in understanding the route of contamination and reveal unsuspected problems of environmental origin. After identifying the *P. aeruginosa* outbreak, a HAI surveillance program based on the National Nosocomial Infections Surveillance (NNIS) System protocol was started in the Hospital [Sodano et al., 2004].

In the assessment of the preventable proportion of infections one approach consists in integrating clonality assessment with a unit-based surveillance protocol intended for continuous surveillance, in which denominator data (patient-days) are collected for the entire unit. Although indicators generated by such a "first-level" surveillance are not suitable for ICU benchmarking of quality of care in terms of infection control, they are appropriate for the follow-up of infections within the same unit and for regional, national and international investigation of trends for pathogen-specific infection rates. This approach has been used in a study conducted with the main aim to investigate the epidemiological impact of *A. baumannii* HAI in a Sicilian ICU and to estimate the preventable proportion of *Acinetobacter* infections, i.e., those resulting from cross-transmission [Agodi et al., 2006]. *A. baumannii* is an increasingly important nosocomial pathogen. Although multiresistant *A. baumannii* strains have been related to outbreak situations, they are now substantially associated to infections endemic to hospitals. This organism is able to survive in the hospital environment for long periods, and several studies have emphasized the importance of environmental cleaning in controlling *A. baumannii* cross-transmission. Cross-transmission could also result from the airborne route as well as from contact with patients. Patients without signs or symptoms of infection and staff could be colonized, and direct contact with colonized skin may be a route of transmission among patients or from staff to patients [Barbolla et al., 2008]. The study was conducted between November 2001 and February 2004. All 665 patients admitted to the combined surgical and medical ICU of the Azienda Ospedaliera S. Giovanni di Dio, in Agrigento (Sicily, Italy) were enrolled into the laboratory-based alert surveillance, performed by trained personnel using the unit-based protocol of the Hospitals in Europe Link for Infection Control through Surveillance [HELICS, 2004]. Infection data were collected for each episode of *Acinetobacter* infection with onset within the surveillance period. The number of new admissions and the number of patient-days for patients staying >2 days in the ICU were also collected. In this study, there were 3.0 new *Acinetobacter* infections *per* 100 admissions to the ICU. Of these, 65% were ICU-acquired pneumonia, 25% were UTIs, and 10% were bloodstream infections. The incidence rate, adjusted by the number of patient-days, was 3.5 infections *per* 1000 patient-days. Molecular typing by PFGE of *Apa*I-digested genomic DNA was performed as described previously [Marroni et al., 2004]. Interpretation of genomic relatedness was performed using well-established criteria [Tenover et al., 1995]. The presence of two indistinguishable strains in two patients was considered to represent one episode of cross-transmission. In general, the number of cross-transmissions that occurred in a ward was calculated by subtracting 1 from the number of indistinguishable strains in different patients [Weist et al., 2002]. Macrorestriction analysis of the *Acinetobacter* isolates identified eight unrelated PFGE types: six were single patterns associated with sporadic isolates; the remaining two were associated with cross-transmission of infection. There were 14 episodes of cross-transmission, accounting for 66.7% of all *A. baumannii* infections.

The proportion of potentially preventable HAIs has been addressed by a systematic review of the published literature describing multi-modal intervention studies and transmission studies performed during the last decade [Harbarth et al., 2003]. It was concluded that > 20% of all HAI are probably avoidable, but that further research into the feasibility and cost effectiveness of prevention is required. Few studies have addressed the issue of estimating the preventable proportion of HAI under routine conditions [Harbarth et al., 2003; Gastmeier P. 2004], and there are even fewer reports concerning ICU-acquired infections caused by *Acinetobacter* spp. in Italy [Villari et al., 1999; Zarrilli et al., 2004]. Although indicators generated by such a 'first-level' surveillance are not suitable for ICU benchmarking of quality of care in terms of infection control, they are appropriate for the follow-up of infections within the same unit and for regional, national and international investigation of trends for pathogen-specific infection rates [HELICS, 2004]. This surveillance study estimated the preventable proportion of *A. baumannii* HAI in the ICU as 66.7%. Thus, exogenous transmission may be considered as a major infection control problem, even in a ward with low baseline rates, indicating that there is still scope for improvement and that the preventive potential is even higher than the figure of 20% determined previously [Harbarth et al., 2003]. Even in an endemic setting with low infection rates, *A. baumannii* spread occurs mainly as a result of cross-infection problems that require appropriate surveillance and infection control policies [Gastmeier P. 2004]. Although the present study was not designed to identify risk-factors, there was no adequate infection control program at the time of the study. Cross-transmission may have occurred via inadequate decontamination of patient-care equipment [Bergogne-Berezin et al., 1996; Herruzo et al., 2004], poor hand hygiene and insufficient routine cleaning of clinical areas [Webster et al., 1998]. Feedback of surveillance data to healthcare personnel, including molecular typing data of bacterial isolates and their associated antibiotic resistance genes, is essential to prevent horizontal transmission [Scheckler et al., 1998; Gaynes et al., 2001]. A molecular-based approach to the control of *Acinetobacter* HAI would provide an insight into the population dynamics of bacterial circulation in the hospital setting, and would allow the design of evidence-based strategies to decrease specific infection rates to the irreducible minimum.

An alternative comprehensive approach integrating patient-based surveillance data, intended for advanced risk-adjusted comparison of infection rates between ICUs, with molecular typing data has been adopted in a recent study in order to investigate the clonality patterns sustaining the endemic *versus* the epidemic mode of transmission for acquisition of the three emerging multiresistant pathogens, *P. aeruginosa*, *A. baumannii* and *S. maltophilia* [Agodi et al., 2007; Barchitta et al., 2008].

A six-months surveillance prospective survey, in accordance with the HELICS protocol [HELICS, 2004], was performed from January to July 2004 at the Azienda Ospedaliera Cannizzaro in Catania (Sicily, Italy). The surveillance methodology was described in greater detail elsewhere [Agodi et al., 2007]. The study focused on three different epidemiological patterns of *P. aeruginosa*, *A. baumannii* and *S. maltophilia* acquisition: i) carriage on admission, ii) colonization of sterile sites and iii) infection during ICU stay. Standard definitions of carriage, colonization and HAI were used [Bertrand et al., 2001; HELICS, 2004; Agodi et al., 2007].

During the study period, 121 patients were enrolled in the ICU surveillance study. Carriage of *P. aeruginosa* upon admission occurred in 1.6 *per* 100 patients. No episode of *A. baumannii* or *S. maltophilia* carriage upon admission was identified. The overall ICU-acquired colonization rate was 54.5 *per* 100 patients and the incidence density was 30.5 *per* 1000 patient-days. The overall ICU-acquired infection rate was 61.1 *per* 100 patients and the incidence density was 34.2 *per* 1000 patient-days.

Molecular typing by PFGE of the digested genomic DNA was performed using different protocols for each bacterial species as previously described [Grothues et al., 1988; Denton et al., 1998; Agodi et al., 2007]. Definition of a cross-transmission episode was based both on the pathogens' PFGE pattern and the patient time of stay in the ward: a cross-transmission episode was assumed when two patients had indistinguishable isolates [Weist et al., 2002] and were treated in the ICU during intervals that overlapped or were no more than seven days apart [Halwani et al., 2006].

Macrorestriction analysis of *P. aeruginosa* isolates led to the identification of eighteen unrelated PFGE-types: one was the major clone responsible for the epidemic spread of *P. aeruginosa* (60.8% of isolates); six were associated with cross-transmission of infection and/or colonization; and the remaining PFGE-types were associated with sporadic strains [Agodi et al., 2007]. Among the *A. baumannii* isolates an unique PFGE-type was identified and among the *S. maltophilia* isolates four distinct clones, all associated with cross-transmission of infection and/or colonization, were identified.

Infections that seem to be most amenable to control measures are those that result from transmission between patients [Grundmann et al., 2005]. Until now, few studies have focused on cross-transmission of nosocomial pathogens in ICU patients under normal conditions. The proportion of nosocomial HAIs as a result of cross-transmission in this study accounted for 50% of the total number of ICU-acquired infections, with an incidence rate of 17.1 *per* 1000 patient-days, the highest figures reported so far by analogous studies [Weist et al., 2002; Grundmann et al., 2005; Halwani et al., 2007]. When cross-colonization was included the impact of cross-transmission was at least 44.3%. The overall risk of cross-transmission of infection and colonization was 28.6 *per* 1000 patient-days. In general, the estimated proportion of cases resulting from transmission may vary depending on the occurrence of outbreaks in the period of study [Mikolajczyk et al., 2007]. Our results provided evidence for the epidemic spread of the three pathogens in the ICU, thus confirming cross-transmission as a common mechanism of acquisition of resistant *P. aeruginosa*, *Acinetobacter* spp. and *S. maltophilia*. For each microrganism the specific epidemic curve was plotted to give a visual representation of the trend of infection and of colonization events over the time period. The curves suggest the occurrence of three simultaneous outbreaks. The shape of each curve, containing two peaks, suggests a propagated or progressive source mode of epidemic transmission, reflective of the number of cases caused by person-to-person contact, until control measures are implemented. Outlier analysis, that is the study of cases that stand apart from the overall pattern, led to identification of potential sources for the three outbreaks: a patient admitted on January 9 colonized both by *P. aeruginosa* clone A and *S. maltophilia* clone C and a patient who became colonized in ICU by *A. baumannii*. Thus, colonization was confirmed to represent not only a considerable element of the bacterial load within the ICU but also a continuous potential source of cross-transmission. Patients colonized at admission can introduce the pathogen into hospital units. If screened at admission, these patients can be detected and isolated, thus reducing the risk of transmission for others. Such active screening of all or just high-risk patients is standard procedure in some settings but not in others. Anyway, wherever cross-transmission is an indicator of poor quality of care, infection control policies should be improved.

Elucidation of the risk factors associated with the acquisition of *P. aeruginosa, A. baumannii* and *S. maltophilia* has been an area of active research for clinicians and epidemiologists around the world. A recent review of the available international literature concluded that the spread of these microrganisms is related to a large number of variables [Falagas et al., 2006]. The main purpose of our study was to investigate the patients' risk profile for acquiring cross transmitted infection by the three emerging pathogens in order to develop a better understanding of their epidemiology and to suggest the most appropriate strategies to minimize their spread. In order to identify risk factors for acquiring cross transmitted infection a case-control study was designed: case patients were those involved in an episode of cross-transmission (with undistinguishable strains) while control patients were those infected by sporadic strains and/or those without any infection. Univariate analysis showed that cross-transmission of infection was significantly related to surgical procedure, to length of the mechanical ventilation, central venous catheterization and urinary catheterization. Artificial ventilation is an established risk factor for cross-transmission and it has been suggested that a longer patients' time at risk increases the chance of infection [Halwani et al., 2007; van der Kooi et al., 2007]. In this ICU, as we have previously reported, the ventilator-associated pneumonia rate and the ventilator utilization ratio were both considerably high [Agodi et al., 2007]. More studies are necessary to identify risk factors for HAI in surgery patients admitted to the ICU and to find new strategies to diminish infection rates in this subgroup of patients [Nan et al., 2005].

Conclusion

Surveillance systems for the epidemiological investigation of HAI cross-transmission have become increasingly more complex.

The present survey of investigations on cross-transmission of HAI illustrates the adoption of such methodological approaches, highlighting for each of them the lesson learned. Integrating laboratory data with prospective epidemiological studies does provide both patient rates of infections and microrganism clonality data, leading to the construction of appropriate indicators of the epidemiological *scenario* of cross-tranmission of HAI. These findings provide a framework for further investigation of the role of alert pathogens and/or high-risk clones together with patients' risk factor profiles for appropriate design of effective control strategies especially addressed to ICU patients.

References

Agodi, A. (2000). Sistemi di tipizzazione epidemiologica dei microrganismi responsabili di infezioni in ospedale: uso e valutazione. *Ann. Ig, 12* (Suppl 2): 41 – 46.

Agodi, A. & Pasquarella, C. (2000). Sorveglianza delle infezioni ospedaliere: revisione della letteratura in una prospettiva storica. *Ann. Ig, 12* (Suppl. 2): 23 - 32.

Agodi, A., Zarrilli, R., Barchitta, M., Anzaldi, A., Di Popolo, A., Mattaliano, A., Ghiraldi, E. & Travali, S. (2006). Alert-surveillance of ICU-acquired *Acinetobacter* infections in a Sicilian hospital. *Clin Microbiol Infect, 12*, 241–247.

Agodi, A., Barchitta, M., Cipresso, R., Giaquinta, L., Romeo, MA. & Denaro, C. (2007). *Pseudomonas aeruginosa* carriage, colonization, and infection in ICU patients. *Intensive Care Med, 33*, 1155-1161.

Barbolla, R. E, Centro´n, D, Maimone, S, Rospide, F, Salgueira, C, Altclas, J. & Catalano, M. (2008). Molecular epidemiology of *Acinetobacter baumannii* spread in an adult intensive care unit under an endemic setting. *Am J Infect Control, 36*, 444-52.

Barchitta, M., Cipresso, R., Giaquinta, L., Romeo, M. A., Denaro, C. & Pennisi, C., Agodi, A. (2008). Acquisition and spread of *Acinetobacter baumannii* and *Stenotrophomonas maltophilia* in intensive care patients. *Int J Hyg Environ Health,* Sep *2*.

Bergogne-Berezin, E. & Towner, K. J. (1996). *Acinetobacter* spp. as nosocomial pathogens: Microbiological, clinical, and epidemiological features. *Clin Microbiol Rev 9*, 148–165.

Bertrand, X., Thouverez, M., Talon, D., Boillot, A., Capellier, G., Floriot, C. & Helias, J. P. (2001). Endemicity, molecular diversity and colonisation routes of *Pseudomonas aeruginosa* in intensive care units. *Intensive Care Med, 27*, 1263-1268.

Denton, M., Todd, N. J., Kerr, K. G., Hawkey, P. M. & Littlewood, J. M. (1998). Molecular Epidemiology of *Stenotrophomonas maltophilia* isolated from Clinical Specimens from Patients with Cystic Fibrosis and Associated Environmental Samples. *J Clin Microbiol, 36*, 1953–1958.

Falagas, M. E. & Kopterides, P. (2006). Risk factors for the isolation of multi-drug-resistant *Acinetobacter baumannii* and *Pseudomonas aeruginosa*: a systematic review of the literature. *J Hosp Infect, 64*, 7-15.

Gastmeier, P. (2004). Nosocomial infection surveillance and control policies. *Curr Opin Infect Dis, 17*, 295-301.

Gaynes, R., Richards, C. & Edwards, J. et al. (2001). Feeding back surveillance data to prevent hospital-acquired infections. *Emerg Inf Dis, 7*, 295-298.

Grothues, D., Koopmann, U., Van der Hardt, H. & Tummler, B. (1988). Genome fingerprinting of *Pseudomonas aeruginosa* indicates colonization of cystic fibrosis siblings with closely related strains. *J Clin Microbiol*, 26, 115-123.

Grundmann, H., Barwolff, S. & Tami, A. *et al.* (2005). How many infections are caused by patient-to-patient transmission in intensive care units? *Crit Care Med, 33*, 946-951.

Halwani, M., Solaymani-Dodaran, M., Grundmann, H., Coupland, C. & Slack, R. (2006). Cross-transmission of nosocomial pathogens in an adult intensive care unit: incidence and risk factors. *J Hosp Infect, 63*, 39-46.

Harbarth, S., Sax, H. & Gastmeier, P. (2003). The preventable proportion on nosocomial infections: an overview of published reports. *J Hosp Infect, 54*, 258-266.

Herruzo, R., de la Cruz, J., Fernández-Aceñero, M. J. & Garcia-Caballero, J. (2004). Two consecutive outbreaks of *Acinetobacter baumanii 1-a* in a burn Intensive Care Unit for adults. *Burns*, 30, 419–423.

Hospital In Europe Link For Infection Control Through Surveillance (HELICS). Surveillance of Nosocomial Infections in Intensive Care Units. Protocol Version 6.1, September 2004, [Http://Helics.Univ-Lyon1.Fr/].

Kayabas, U., Bayraktar, M., Otlu, B., Ugras, M., Ersoy, Y., Bayindir, Y. & Durmaz, R. (2008). An outbreak of *Pseudomonas aeruginosa* because of inadequate disinfection procedures in a urology unit: A pulsed field gel electrophoresis-based epidemiologic study. *Am J Infect Control*, *36*, 33-8.

Kayabas, U., Bayraktar, M., Otlu, B., Ugras, M., Ersoy, Y., Bayindir, Y, & Durmaz, R. (2008). An outbreak of *Pseudomonas aeruginosa* because of inadequate disinfection procedures in a urology unit: A pulsed field gel electrophoresis-based epidemiologic study. *Am J Infect Control*, *36*, 33-8.

Koeleman, J. G., Stoof, J., van der Bijl, M. W., Vanderbroucke-Grauls, C. M. J. E. & Savelkou, P. H. M. (2001). Identification of epidemic strains of *Acinetobacter baumanni* by integrase gene PCR. *J Clin Microbiol*, *39*, 8-13.

Marroni, M., Pasquarella, C., Agodi, A., *et al.* (2004). Clonal spread of *Acinetobacter baumannii* in a general intensive care unit. *Ann Ig*, *16*, 95-102

Mikolajczyk, R. T., Sagel, U., Bornemann, R., Kramer, A. & Kretzschmar, M. A. (2007). statistical method for estimating the proportion of cases resulting from cross-transmission of multi-resistant pathogens in an intensive care unit. *J Hosp Infect*, *65*, 149-155.

Nan, D. N., Fernández-Ayala, M., Fariñas-Alvarez, C., Mons, R., Ortega, F. J., González-Macías, J. & Fariñas, M. C. (2005). Nosocomial infection after lung surgery: incidence and risk factors. *Chest*, *128*, 2647-52.

Renders, N., Romling, Y., Verbrugh, H. & van Belkum, A. (1996). Comparative typing of Pseudomonas aeruginosa by random amplification of polymorphic DNA or pulsed-field gel electrophoresis of DNA macrorestriction fragments. *J Clin Microbiol*, *34*, 3190-5.

Scheckler, W. E., Brimhall, D. & Buck, A. S, *et al.* (1998). Requirements for infrastructure and essential activities of infection control and epidemiology in hospitals: a consensus panel report. *Am J Infect Control*, *26*, 47–60.

Sehulster, L. M., Chinn, R. Y. W. & Arduino, M. J. *et al.* (2004). Guidelines for environmental infection control in health-care facilities. Recommendations from CDC and the Healthcare Infection Control Practices Advisory Committee (HICPAC). Chicago IL; American Society for Healthcare Engineering/American Hospital Association;.

Sodano, L., Agodi, A., Barchitta, M., Musumeci, F., Menichetti, A., Bellocchi, P., Consolo, R. & Coco, G. (2004). Nosocomial infections in heart surgery patients: active surveillance in two italian hospitals. *Ann Ig*, *16*, 735-743.

Tenover, F., Arbeit, R. & Goering, R. (1997). How to select and interpret molecular strain typing methods for epidemiological studies of bacterial infections: a review for healthcare epidemiologists. *Infect Control Hosp Epidemiol*, *18*, 426-439.

van der Kooi, T. I. I., de Boer, A. S., Manniën, J. & Wille, J. C, (2007). MT Beaumont, BW Mooi, van den Hof S. Incidence and risk factors of device-associated infections and associated mortality at the intensive care in the Dutch surveillance system. *Intensive Care Med*, *33*, 271–278.

Villari, P., Iacuzio, L. & Vozzella, E. A, Bosco, U. (1999). Unusual genetic heterogeneity of *Acinetobacter baumanni* isolates in a university hospital in Italy. *Am. J. Infect. Control*, *27*, 247-253.

Webster, C. A., Crowe, M., Humphreys, H. & Towner, K. J. (1998). Surveillance of an adult intensive care unit for long-term persistence of a multi-resistant strain of *Acinetobacter baumannii. Eur J Clin Microbiol Infect Dis*, *17*, 171-6.

Weist, K., Pollege, K., Schultz, I., Ruden, H. & Gastmeier, P. (2002). How many nosocomial infections are associated with cross-transmission? A prospective cohort study in a surgical intensive care unit. *Infect Control Hosp Epidemiol*, *23*, 127-132.

Zarrilli, R., Crispino, M. & Bagattini, M. *et al*. (2004). Molecular epidemiology of sequential outbreaks of *Acinetobacter baumannii* in an intensive care unit shows the emergence of carbapenem resistance. *J Clin Microbiol, 42*, 946-953.

In: Cross Infections: Types, Causes and Prevention
Editors: Jin Dong and Xun Liang

ISBN: 978-1-60741-467-4
© 2009 Nova Science Publishers, Inc.

Chapter IX

Mycobacterium Avium-Intracellulare Infection during HIV Disease: Persisting Problems*

Roberto Manfredi[1]
Department of Infectious Diseases, University of Bologna,
S. Orsola-Malpighi Hospital, Bologna, Italy

Abstract

Still in the era of potent, combined antiretroviral therapy, late recognition of HIV disease or lack of sufficient immune recovery pose HIV-infected patients at risk to develop opportunistic infections by atypical mycobacteria, which are environmental organisms commonly retrieved in soil and superficial waters. Among these microorganisms, the most frequent is represented by Mycobacterium avium-intracellulare (Mycobacterium avium-intracellulare complex, or MAC). Health care professionals who face HIV-infected patients should suspect disseminated mycobacterial disease when a deep immunodeficiency is present, as represented by a CD4+ lymphocyte count below 50-100 cells/μL, and often systemic, non-specific signs and symptoms, and associated non-specific laboratory abnormalities. Mycobacterial culture of peripheral blood is a reliable technique for diagnosing disseminated disease. A set of two cultures may identify over 95% of cases of Mycobacterium avium-intracellulare bacteremia. Microscopical examination (Ziehl-Nielsen stain and comparable techniques), and culture biopsies from other normally sterile body sites (i.e. bone marrow, lymph nodes, or liver), also may be useful to pose a diagnosis of AIDS-related mycobacterial disease. Among drugs active against atypical mycobacteria, besides some anti-tubercular compound, the rifampicin derivative rifabutin, and the novel fluoroquinolones, the availability of macrolides greatly

* A version of this chapter was also published in *AIDS-Related Opportunistic Infections,* edited by Claudia Galanda published by Nova Science Publishers, Inc. It was submitted for appropriate modifications in an effort to encourage wider dissemination of research.

[1]Correspondence:Roberto Manfredi, MD, Associate Professor of Infectious Diseases, Universiy of Bologna, c/o Infectious Diseases, S. Orsola Hospital, Via Massarenti 11, I-40138 Bologna, Italy, Telephone: +39-051-6363355, Telefax: +39-051-343500, E-mail: Roberto.manfredi@unibo.it

contributed to improve both prophylaxis and treatment outcome of disseminated mycobacteriosis complicating the course of AIDS. Although multiple questions remain about which regimens are optimal, general recommendations can be expressed on the ground of existing evidences. Treatment should begin with associated clarithromycin (or azithromycin), plus ethambutol and rifabutin (with the rifabutin dosing depending on other concomitant medications that might result in drug-drug interactions). A combined three-drug regimen is preferred for patients who cannot be prescribed an effective antiretroviral regimen immediately. Patients with a CD4+ lymphocyte count below 50 cells/μL who do not have clinical evidence of active mycobacterial disease, should receive a primary prophylaxis with either clarithromycin or azithromycin; the latter could be coadministered rifabutin. Anti-mycobacterial prophylaxis may be discontinued in patients without a history of recognized mycobacterial disease, whose CD4+ lymphocyte count remains above 100 cells/μL, for at least three months while on combined antiretroviral therapy. With regard to subjects on secondary antimycobacterial prophylaxis, in appears safe to discontinue it when a sustained CD4+ lymphocyte count exceeds at least 100 cells/μL for at least 3-6 consecutive months, during a concurrent, effective antiretroviral regimen.

Keywords: HIV disease, opportunistic infections, combined antiretroviral therapy, *Mycobacterium avium-intracellula*re, diagnosis, treatment, prophylaxis

Introduction

Mycobacterium avium-intracellulara complex (MAC) consists of several related species of mycobacteria that are ubiquitous in the environment (especially soil, dust, and superficial waters). MAC is an infrequent cause of human disease in individuals with normal immune defence. On the other hand, in deeply immunocompromised patients, such as those with advanced HIV infection and AIDS, MAC still represent common and serious opportunistic infections [1, 2]. Among HIV-infected subjects followed in the pre-antiretroviral therapy era, disseminated MAC has historically occurred especially when the CD4+ T-lymphocyte count dropped at values below 50 cells/μL [1, 2]. Colonization of the airways (and also the gastrointestinal tract) by MAC can occur without evident morbidity; however, MAC colonization of these sites points out that the relevant patients are at increased risk for developing disseminated MAC infection [3]. The potent, combination antiretroviral therapies (cART) introduced since mid-1996 (12 years go), have been associated with a significant reduction in AIDS-related mortality, days of hospitalization, and the incidence of novel or recurring opportunism, including MAC disease [4]. However, there have been numerous reports of atypical clinical presentations of MAC, just since the introduction of cART [5-10], so that differential diagnosis remains difficult still in the third millennium. The diagnosis can pose challenges to the clinician because isolation of these organisms is often difficult. In addition, both active disease and airway colonization occur in individuals with structural defects or previous or concurrent illnessess, adding further confusion for health caregivers. Furthermore, these organisms are frequently contaminants, leading to false-positive diagnoses in patients with other active diseases. The treatment of non-tuberculoius atypical mycobacterial infections is as difficult as establishing a correct diagnosis because therapy is often prolonged, difficult to tolerate, and frequently ineffective. Given these challenges, especially in the face of a progressive increase in the prevalence of this disease, clinicians should be familiar with these emerging disorders, whose incidence may increase among immunocompromised patients other than those with HIV/AIDS [1]. There is convincing evidence that an effective treatment of disseminated MAC infection improves both survival and quality of life of patients living with HIV infection and AIDS [11]. Whether MAC can be eradicated once disseminated infection has occurred is still uncertain, but some evidences suggest that secondary prophylaxis may be discontinued in patients who have had sustained immunologic recovery thanks to an effective cART [12-14]. The treatment regimen for disseminated MAC occurring during HIV infection, should include at least two active drugs, in order to ensure efficacy and prevent the emerging of microbial resistance. The most efficacious drugs for MAC treatment are the newer macrolide antibiotics, represented by clarithromycin and azithromycin [15-17]. The preferred treatment regimen should include one of these last two macrolides, together with ethambutol and/or rifabutin (a rifampicin derivative with improved activity against MAC) [18-21]. Clarithromycin, azithromycin, or rifabutin should be administered as a primary or secondary prophylaxis to prevent MAC disease or MAC relapse in all HIV-infected patients with a CD4+ lymphocyte count persistingly under 50 cells/μL, despite cART co-administration [22-25].

Microbiological and Epidemiological Notes

The group of MAC organisms consists of *M. avium-intracellulare*, and other species of *Mycobacterium* that have not been classified in particular. In the past, it was difficult to distinguish *M. avium* from *M. intracellulare*, as the laboratory assay relied on organism serotyping. Therefore, it was common to refer to them as *M avium-intracellulare*. Of the 28 known seroagglutination MAC types, types 1 to 6, types 8 to 11, and type 21 are classified as *M. avium*; type 7, types 12 to 20, and type 25 are classified as *M. intracellulare*; while types 22 to 24 and types 26 to 28 have not been classified until now [26]. Using DNA probe techniques, it is now possible to rapidly identify *M. avium* and *M. intracellulare* [27]. However, in most cases of AIDS-related disease, disseminated MAC infection is caused by *M. avium* species, and from a therapeutic and prophylactic point of view there is no significant difference. MAC strains may vary in their intrinsic pathogenicity, which may explain why *M. avium* serotypes 4 and 8 are the most common organisms to infect immunocompromised patients suffering from AIDS [28, 29]. Some identified biological markers of the pathogenicity of the MAC organisms include the presence of plasmid, antibiotic susceptibility patterns, multilocus enzyme electrophoretic profiles, and restriction fragment length polymorphism patterns [30-32]. Superficial water, soil and dust have been implicated as possible environmental sources of MAC for HIV-infected patients (as well as for the general population). Duiring a documented nosocomial outbreak, the hospital water supply was the ascertained origin of a well defined MAC strain, with showed the same restriction fragment length polymorphism profile as that infecting a group of hospitalized AIDS persons with AIDS [33]. Furthermore, no apparent differences have been observed in the frequency of disseminated MAC infection according to age, gender, race, geographic areas, the different exposure to HIV infection transmission, antiretroviral therapy selection, and initial AIDS-defining conditions [34].

Pathogenesis and Pathologic Features

The mechanisms of spread and acquisition of disseminated MAC infection are still incompletely understood. As such, not all non-tuberculous mycobacterial isolates represent true infections, since they may be trivial colonization or contamination. Currenly available data support the hypothesis that MAC disease results from recent environmental transmission of MAC through either the respiratory tract or the gastroenteric tract, rather than from a reactivation of latent MAC infection. However, after acquiring a clinically-evident MAC infection, the eventual, underlying immunodeficiency becomes the most relevant factor which supports the eventual disease recurrences during the follow-up; it was true especially before the cART era, but it remains possible still 12 years after the introduction of cART. As anticipated, among HIV-infected patients with a primary disease manifestation, the occurrence of MAC dissemination does not vary among age groups [34]. Therefore, should reactivation of latent infection was the mechanism of acquisition, the incidence of dissemination would expected to increase with age, much like in tuberculosis (which is known to be primarily caused by reactivation of latent infection). From an immunological point of view, the risk of developing HIV-associated MAC infection is inversely related with the absolute CD4+ lymphocyte count. In one observational study, the measured one-year incidence of MAC bacteremia was 3% for patients with a CD4+ count in the 100-199 cells/μL range, as compared with 39% for patients with a CD4+ count under 10 cells/μL [2]. The same study also underlined that individuals with a far advanced HIV disease had a linear increase in the risk of developing MAC bacteremia over time, and the risk of developing disseminated MAC infection for patients surviving for 30 months after being diagnosed with AIDS was around 50% [2]. Other observational studies and prophylaxis trials added several, consistent findings: the risk of development of disseminated MAC disease ranged from 30% to 50% of patients with a CD4+ lymphocyte counts below 50 cells/μL, in the absence of specific antimicrobial prophylaxis [1, 23, 25]. In particular, the difficulty to mount a retrievable antibody response to MAC in HIV-infected patients with disseminated MAC infection may also suggests a recent primary infection, because deeply immunocompromised HIV-infected patients lack the ability to establish antibody responses to multiple, primary infections [35, 36]. Furthermore, literature reports of MAC colonization of the respiratory or gastroenteric tract preceding the occurrence of disseminated MAC infection suggest that the organism is first acquired from the environment and subsequently disseminated, when a severe underlying immunosuppression is of concern [3, 37]. Finally, the incidence of disseminated MAC disease among patients with AIDS substantially exceeds the frequency of MAC infection in the general population, as determined by population studies, and confirmed by MAC-specific skin testing, too [38]. As anticipated, MAC dissemination requires a susceptible host. By the year 1984, only 37 cases of disseminated MAC infection in non-HIV-infected humans were reported, the majority of them occurring in patients with identifiable, severe immunological deficiencies [39]. In the non-HIV-infected population, MAC infection generally cause localized lesions: cervical lymphadenitis in children, a slowly progressive fibrocavitary pulmonary disease in middle-aged men with a chronic, underlying lung disease (i.e. chronic obstructive pulmonary disease or COPD, lung emphysema, bronchiectasis, pulmonary fibrosis, and pneumoconiosis), or localized bronchiectasis in women who have a narrow anteroposterior chest diameter, pectus excavatum, scoliosis, or mitral valve prolapse and associated conditions (i.e. Marfan's syndrome) [40, 41]. The blunted immune response and the lack of local and systemic inflammatory reaction typical of patients with AIDS and a deep HIV-related immunodeficiency who develop disseminated MAC disease is consistent with the hypothesis that the key immunologic defects associated with dissemination are defective monocyte-macrophage killing of phagocytized MAC and a defective cytokine network response, including abnormally low levels of tumor necrosis factor (TNF), interferon-gamma, and interleukin-12 [42-46]. As a result of this extremely permissive immunological environment, MAC infection becomes widespread in extremely immunosuppressed HIV-infected patients, and it was the case of the majority of subjects suffering from MAC disease during the pre-cART era (i.e. before mid-nineties). In the majority of autopsy examinations performed in these patients who died of these opportunistic infections in the pre-cART era, MAC organisms have been isolated from lymph nodes, spleen, liver, lung, adrenal glands, gastrointestinal tract (colon), kidney, and bone marrow, but the multivisceral dissemination has virtually no limits, and may involve all body organs and sites. In fact, the magnitude of mycobacteremia has been estimated to be as high as 10,000 organisms/μL of blood, the equivalent of 10 billion organisms per gram of bone marrow, spleen, lymph node, and liver tissue obtained at necropsy examination [47]. Not surprisingly, the histopathologic examination of liver, spleen, bone marrow, or gut from patients with AIDS-related disseminated MAC disease shows a high-grade widespread infection, together with a lack (or a reduced) inflammatory infiltrate or tissue necrosis. In contrast, histopathologic examination of tissue from patients with AIDS who have localized, non-disseminated MAC infection demonstrates marked inflammatory reaction and tissue destruction similar to the histopathologic findings observed in association with non-HIV-associated MAC or mycobacterial lung or lymph node infection. On the other hand, at the time of cART availability, the rapid recovery of immune defences obtained thanks to the elevated and prompt antiviral activity of available anti-HIV compounds, is the basis of the so-called immune-reconstitution syndrome, which is more prominent just in patients with a prior-latent, or a recently acquired MAC infection (see below).

Clinical Presentation

As anticipated, disseminated non-tuberculous mycobacterial disease is not uncommon when advanced HIV infection is of concern. Prior to effective antiretroviral therapy (cART), nearly 40% of patients with CD4+ lymphocyte counts less than 10 50 cells/μL developed disseminated disease within one year of observation. The risk for disseminated MAC infection increases with progressively lower CD4+ lymphocyte counts. This AIDS-defining disease typically occurs when CD4+ lymphocyte counts are below 25 cells/μL, but patients with CD4+ counts less than 50-100 cells/μL are at elevated risk. Usually, a systemic illness caused by atypical mycobacteria (MAC) occurs as a severe, life-threatening opportunistic infection in patients with advanced HIV infection or AIDS, who has a CD4+ lymphocyte count under 50-100 cells/μL. Subjects who suffer from a disseminated MAC infection frequently show non-specific signs and symptoms, and multiple, but non-specific laboratory abnormalities. In many instances, a progressive worsening of constitutional symptoms may reflect a disseminated MAC infection, and this aspect can be incorrectly referred to the progression of HIV disease itself or multiple, HIV-related illnesses. Patients affected by MAC disease most commonly report persistent fever (not responding to a broad-spectrum empiric antibiotic therapy), remarkable night sweats, asthenia, extreme fatigue, anorexia, and weight loss up to cachexia (the so-called wasting syndrome). Aspecific abdominal pain or irregular-chronic diarrhea, may result from the involvement of retroperitoneal lymph nodes or gastroenteric mucosa, respectively, by disseminated MAC disease A notable hepatosplenomegaly and a diffuse lymphadenopathy, may also complete the clinical picture. Intraabdominal lymphadenopathy is frequent, as demonstrated using abdominal computed tomography (CT) in 14 of 17 patients with disseminated MAC infection [48], and may be easily detected by abdominal ultrasonographic studies. From a laboratory point of view, pancytopenia (represented by slowly progressing anemia, leukopenia, and thrombocytopenia), is the most common occurrence, while elevated serum alkaline phosphatase and lactic dehydrogenase levels, or low albumin levels have been also reported frequently. In a prospective, observational survey of MAC bacteremia conducted at a single-centre United States Hospital during the pre-cART era, the authors interviewed patients with a CD4+ lymphocyte count lower than 50 cells/μL regarding signs and symptoms, and evaluated the laboratory workup conducted as part of the diagnostic evaluation for disseminated MAC infection [49]. A history of fever lasting for more than one month, a hematocrit under 30%, or serum albumin levels below 3.0 g/dL, proved affordable predictors of MAC bacteremia. On the other hand, severe fatigue, diarrhea, weight loss, neutropenia, and thrombocytopenia did not seem to play a significant role in discriminating between patients who were subsequently found to have MAC-positive blood cultures, and those who were culture-negative for MAC, in an univariate analysis [49]. More unusual manifestations of viceral MAC infection include a broad spectrum of organic-systemic localizations, including oral (palatal and gingival) ulcerations, septic arthritis, osteomyelitis, endophthalmitis, pericarditis, and massive gastrointestinal bleeding [50-54]. Non-tuberculous mycobacterial pulmonary localization is almost always associated with symptoms such as chronic or recurring cough, sputum production, and exertional dyspnea. Hemoptysis, although uncommon, can occur (thus entering a frank tuberculosis in the differential diagnosis). However, also in these patients with a suspected respiratory localization, constitutional symptoms such as fever, fatigue, malaise, night sweats, and weight loss occur, and often predominate.

Diagnosis and Microbiological Workup

The diagnosis of disseminated MAC disease frequently poses severe challenges to the clinicians. As stated, MAC are ubiquitous to the environment and may represent contamination rather than actual isolates. Additionally, MAC and other non-tuberculous mycobacteria may colonize the airways of individuals with structural lung abnormalities, or chronic respiratory disorders. As a consequence, recovery of these microorganisms may represent airway colonization, rather than true infection. Therefore, discovery of MAC does not necessarily reflect disease. The diagnosis must be based on a high clinical suspicion that is compatible with symptoms and clinical features. When a respiratory localization is suspected, sputum cultures are not reliable since they are often negative, and bronchoscopic washing (or preferably bronchoalveolar lavage) may be a more useful diagnostic tool. However, in the right clinical setting, a single positive culture from bronchoscopic washing or bronchoalveolar lavage may be considered diagnostic. Tissue specimens obtained from biopsy stiudies (transbronchial lung biopsy, surgical lung biopsy, or excisional biopsy from infected tissues), are also diagnostic if they lead to the isolation of MAC organisms or show granulomatous inflammation on histopathologic examination. In the right clinical setting with highly suspicious clinical and imaging findings, tests in which cultures are negative should be repeated, as isolation of atypical mycobacterios is often difficult. Finally, a true *M. tuberculosis* disease must be excluded in all cases of suspected MAC, especially when pulmonary infiltrates and acid-fast bacillus smear positivity are of concern. With regard to patients with advanced HIV infection, systematic culture search of MAC from peripheral blood is a sensitive and easy method for diagnosing disseminated MAC infection. Mycobacterial blood cultures allow to establish the diagnosis of disseminated MAC disease with a very elevated sensitivity (ranging from 86% to 98% of cases in which disseminated MAC infection was subsequently confirmed at necropsy examination) [55, 56]. While one single blood culture set leads to identify around 90% of HIV-infected patients with MAC bacteremia, the adjunct of a second blood culture increases the identification rate up to 98% [57, 58]. The preferred culture assays are preceded by a lysis of peripheral blood leukocytes, to release intracellular mycobacteria, followed by seeding onto solid media (usually the classic Lowenstein-Jensen agar, or similar mediums), or into radiometric broths of commerce [59, 60]. Using this last radiometric assays, atypical mycobacteria can be detected from blood cultures in as few as 6-12 days, whereas 15-40 days are required with the traditional, solid media. Furthermore, currently available DNA probes and PCR assays can identify and distinguish among MAC species within as few as a two-three hours, after that a sufficient mycobacterial growth has occurred in radiometric broth or on solid media [27, 61]. As known, tissue biopsies obtained from normally sterile body sites also can prove diagnostic. For exemple, simple stains of biopsy specimens obtained from bone marrow, lymph nodes, or liver, may easily demonstrate acid-fast bacilli or a tubercular-like granulomatous lesion, sometimes weeks before positive blood culture results become evident [62, 63]. It is also possible that culture of bone marrow, lymph node, or liver, could be more sensitive compared with blood cultures, especially when a subacute-chronic disease has been already established, and a deep immunodeficiency concurs, as is the case of advanced HIV disease.

Therapeutic Management of MAC Infection in the Setting of HIV Disease

The treatment of disseminated MAC disease is seldom straightforward, especially in the field of HIV infection and AIDS. Diagnostic uncertainty is common, prolonged durations of therapy are frequently needed, and eradication is unlikely whilst underlying immunodeficiency remains present. Moreover, treatment regimens are expensive, and are often poorly tolerated because of frequent side effects, and the expected drug-drug interaction with multiple compounds frequently co-administered to patient living with HIV disease [1]. In some cases, patients with disseminated MAC describe the treatment as being worse than the disease itself. As known, mycobacterial organisms other than tuberculosis (and MAC in particular) are not killed by standard antituberculous drugs except ethambutol (at *in vivo* achievable plasma concentrations). However, based on extensive observational *in vitro* testings, at least 50% of MAC strains can be inhibited by achievable serum levels of a series of antimicrobial drugs, including rifabutin, rifampin, clofazimine, cycloserine, amikacin, ethionamide, azithromycin, clarithromycin, ciprofloxacin, sparfloxacin, and moxifloxacin. Unfortunately, plasma drug levels needed to obtain a complete *in vitro* killing of MAC (the so-called minimum bactericidal concentration, or MBC value) range from 8 to over 32 times compared with minimum inhibitory levels (minimum inhibitor concentration, or MIC value) [64]. While associated antimycobacterial agents have shown *in vitro* inhibitory synergism, a truly bactericidal synergism has been more difficult to be demonstrated [64, 65]. Moreover, in order to ensure *in vivo* bactericidal acitvity, the relevant drugs must penetrate mononuclear cells (especially macrophages) at a suitable concentrations, and must ensure levels capable to pass the bacterial cell wall of MAC organisms. Anyway, some reliable animal models of disseminated MAC infection showed that both single and combination antimycobacterial regimens led to reduced mycobacterial colony counts by several logs, and also improved animal survival [66, 67]. Medical therapy for disseminated MAC disease involves multiple agents, in order to facilitate clearance of organisms, and to minimize the emergence of drug resistance. The cornerstone agents include macrolides, ethambutol, and the rifamycin derivative rifabutin [1]. Three-drug regimens are preferred because of concerns for the development of macrolide resistance. In fact, some last-generation macrolides, in particular clarithromycin and azithromycin, showed very encouraging *in vitro* and *in vivo* efficacy against MAC. A multicenter, randomized, placebo-controlled trial performed in the pre-cART era, assessed clarithromycin monotherapy, in dosages of 500, 1,000, and 2,000 mg (twice daily), in patients with a primary diagnosis of disseminated MAC. The investigators reported a median decrease of over 2 logs in bacterial colony-forming units from blood culture specimens, thus demonstrating a more potent microbiologic effect than had been reported in earlier treatment trials, together with an affordable *in vivo* response [15]. However, a dose-response effect was not observed, but elevated gastrointestinal intolerance occurred with the 2,000-mg twice daily dosage. Although the 1,000-mg twice-daily dosage led to a greater microbiologic response *versus* the 500-mg twice-daily dosing, there was a trend towards an increased mortality in association with the 1,000-mg dosage [15]. When considering that monotherapy regimens were challenged, it was not surprising that drug resistance emerged after 2-3 months of isolated macrolide administration in this trial, affecting around 50% of patients, regardless of used dosages. Daily therapy is strongly recommended in the majority of cases. However, for patients who cannot tolerate daily therapy or those who do not require an aggressive treatment strategy, intermittent (three times-weekly) therapy, may be adequate. As anticipated, macrolides are the most effective agents against NTMB. As such, current guidelines recommend that macrolides be part of all regimens for NTMB infections [1]. Although effective, these agents should not be used as monotherapy to help prevent the risk of resistance. As a consequence, despite a growing evidence that the optimal agent for disseminated MAC therapy may be represented by clarithromycin or azithromycin, the macrolide administration should be "protected", after the combination with other antimycobacterial agents, in order to prevent or at least delay the emergence of microbial resistance, which is parallely associated with clinical deterioration, and a less favorable clinical outcome. A subsequent study confirmed that the 1,000-mg twice-daily dosage of clarithromycin has an adverse effect on survival compared with the 500 mg twice-daily dosing [68]. As anticipated, azithromycin is another macrolide which is fully effective for MAC treatment. In a trial of azithromycin monotherapy, patients with newly diagnosed positive MAC blood cultures received randomized administration of 1 of 2 doses of azithromycin, 600 or 1,200 mg daily. After six weeks, approximately one half of blood cultures were sterile in both groups, with a mean reduction in mycobacteremia of 2 and 1.55 logs, respectively [16]. As a consequence, we can suppose that the antimycobacterial activity of azitrhomycin was similar to that obtained with clarithromycin monotherapy. As already observed with clarithromycin, the higher dosage of azithromycin was related to a higher rate of gastrointestinal intolerance. A number of other antimycobacterial agents has been assessed in several randomized, controlled trials. In one trial performed before the introduction of cART, investigators compared the microbiologic efficacy of four-week monotherapy regimens of rifampin, ethambutol, or clofazimine in patients with previously untreated disseminated MAC [68]: only ethambutol achieved a statistically significant reduction in blood MAC colony-forming units, suggesting that ethambutol might be the most potent of these three compared antimycobacterial agents. A rifampicin derivative, named rifabutin, had been specifically developed for the management of disseminated MAC infection in the immunocompromised patient. In an early (1994) randomized, placebo-controlled trial in which patients with newly diagnosed disseminated MAC disease were blindly assigned to receive clofazimine/ethambutol or clofazimine/ethambutol/rifabutin (at 600 mg/day), approximately half of the patients receiving the rifabutin-containing regimen had a >2 log decrease in blood MAC colony-forming units, or sterilization of the blood, compared with none of those receiving only clofazimine/ethambutol combination [19]. The long-term clinical outcome of combination regimens including both macrolide and non-macrolide agents for treatment of disseminated HIV-associated MAC disease, was confirmed in a randomized multicenter trial published in the year 1996 [11]. This study included 187 patients with ascertained MAC mycobacteremia, who were randomized to receive clarithromycin at 1,000 mg twice daily, rifabutin 300-600 mg once daily, and ethambutol 15 mg/kg/day, or a regimen of ciprofloxacin 750 mg twice daily, rifampin 600 mg once daily, clofazimine 100 mg once daily, and ethambutol 15 mg/kg/day [11] The *in vivo* quantitative antimycobacterial efficacy tested significantly better with the macrolide-containing regimen, as was median patients' survival (8.6 *versus* 5.2 months; $p<.001$). Although multiple investigations contributed with the evidence of positive results, the composition of the optimal treatment regimen for disseminated MAC in patients with HIV disease is still uncertain. Based on the available microbiological and clinical data, a macrolide drug (either clarithromycin or azithromycin), should be part of the regimen. No significant differences in mortality rates was noticed in a randomized, double-blind trial comparing azithromycin at 600 mg once daily with clarithromycin 500 mg orally twice a day, in an ethambutol-based regimen [17]. Evidences coming from a 1995 trial of several clarithromycin-containing regimens suggested that clofazimine compared poorly with ethambutol as a second drug added to clarithromycin [18]. Furthermore, a randomized clinical trial that added clofazimine to clarithromycin plus rifabutin found a greater mortality rate in the clofazimine-containing arm (62% with clofazimine *versus* 38% without clofazimine; $p=.012$) [70]. Another randomized trial which assessed a four-drug, oral antimycobacterial regimen with or without parenteral amikacin showed no clinical benefit associated with amikacin adjunct [71]. A large, open-label, prospective, randomized trial comparing the efficacy and safety of clarithromycin plus ethambutol, rifabutin, or both for the treatment of disseminated MAC was conducted in the year 2003 [20]. Of 203 enrolled patients, 53 received clarithromycin and ethambutol, 50 received clarithromycin and rifabutin, and 57 received all three drugs. A complete microbiologic response (as defined by sterile blood cultures obtained at 12 weeks), was found in 40%, 42%, and 51% of cases, respectively. Notably, a significant improvement in survival was observed in the three-drug arm [20]. Anyway, another randomized, placebo-controlled study which assessed the addition of rifabutin to a regimen of clarithromycin and ethambutol failed in finding differences in the microbiologic response or survival benefit between the two stated arms [21]. Moreover, this last study detected a significant reduction in the development of clarithromycin resistance in the arm containing three drugs (2% *versus* 14%), thus suggesting a possible benefit in the field of microbial resistance, too [21]. Macrolide resistance occurs and typically results from macrolide monotherapy, although the concomitant use of fluoroquinolones has been suggested as an adjunctive supporting cause. Regimens that do not include ethambutol are also associated with the development of drug resistance. Unfortunately, in cases of macrolide resistance, mortality occurs within one year in approximately one third of patients and, nearly half of patients will die within two years [1]. In the immunocompromised host, treatment should be continued for up to 12 months; negative sputum cultures should be obtained in pulmonary localizations. Therefore, the typical duration of treatment may range from 18 to 24 months, but it can be even longer for some individuals, whose immune recovery last longer. Also in the cART era, treatment failure and recurrences of disseminated MAC disease are somewhat common. Patients are considered to be a treatment failure if they have not shown clinical improvements after six months of appropriate treatment, or have not achieved negative sputum culture after 12 months of appropriate therapy (in the event of isolated respiratory tract disease). Treatment failure may be related to treatment non-compliance or intolerance, local anatomic defects (cavitation or bronchiectasis, when lung disease is of concern), or drug resistance (especially to macrolides, as discussed above). Relapses and re-infections are also common, and may not be necessarily related to a rising drug resistance, compared with the underlying patients' immunodeficiency. Treatment failures are unlikely to have a successful course of re-treatment, in the majority of cases. Therefore many authors advocate aggressive treatment initially. Surgical resection may be effective in patients with focal (especially pulmonary) MAC disease, and is considered curative for solitary pulmonary nodules caused by MAC infection.

Antimycobacterial Prophylaxis Guidelines

Since up to 40% of patients with advanced HIV disease are likely to develop disseminated MAC, it makes sense to develop a strategy for preventing this disease in patients at risk (the so-called *primary prophylaxis*). Few specific risk factors, other than a low CD4+ lymphocyte count, have been clearly defined until now. Therefore, any current prophylactic strategy must be applied to the entire population at risk, specifically, patients with HIV infection and a concurrent CD4+ lymphocyte count below 50 cells/μL. Results of combined analysis of two randomized, placebo-controlled trials of rifabutin prophylaxis carried out in the pre-cART era, which included more than 1000 patients with advanced HIV disease, showed that rifabutin at 300 mg/day reduced the incidence of mycobacteremia by around 50% [25]. Interestingly, patients who received rifabutin and subsequently developed mycobacteremia had blood MAC isolates that retained susceptibility to rifabutin. However, neither each single trial, nor their combined analysis, demonstrated that rifabutin significantly reduced mortality. Combined analysis of both trials revealed an increased incidence of fever, fatigue, anemia, elevated alkaline phosphatase levels, and hospitalizations in patients who received placebo compared with those who received rifabutin. Patients assigned to the placebo arm in these last trials, however, tended to have a lower absolute CD4+ cell count, which may have accounted for some of the greater morbidity [25]. A further placebo-controlled study provided the first evidence that MAC prophylaxis could improve survival of patients with late-stage HIV disease. Six hundred and 82 patients with advanced HIV disease were randomly assigned to receive either clarithromycin (500 mg) or placebo twice daily. During a median 10-month follow-up period, only 6% of clarithromycin-treated subjects developed mycobacteremia compared with 16% of placebo-assigned patients (p<.001) [23]. Notably, the median patients' survival time was significantly longer for clarithromycin-assigned patients than for placebo-assigned patients (8.6 *versus* 5.2 months; p=.001). Dose-limiting drug toxicity occurred in 8% of the clarithromycin group, and 6% of the placebo group [23]. A prior trial had already provided even more convincing evidence of the long-term benefit of clarithromycin prophylaxis for MAC in patients with very advanced HIV disease. A total of 1216 patients with a median absolute CD4+ lymphocyte count of 28 cells/μL were randomly assigned to receive rifabutin (300-450 mg/day), clarithromycin (500 mg twice daily), or a combination of these agents [22]. Median follow-up of patients enrolled in this trial was 589 days (over 19 months), longer than in any other MAC prophylaxis trial ever performed; overall survival was approximately 50%. At the conclusion of the trial, deaths in the respective groups were: clarithromycin, 42%; rifabutin, 43%; and the combination, 46% [22]. In an intent-to-treat analysis, only 9% of patients assigned to clarithromycin developed disseminated MAC, compared with 15% assigned to rifabutin (p<.001). The combination of clarithromycin and rifabutin did not act better than clarithromycin alone [22]. Data from previous natural history studies and placebo-controlled prophylaxis trials would predict, in this trial group, a 36% incidence of disseminated MAC at 19 months in the absence of any MAC chemoprophylaxis [22]. Therefore, based on these last evidences, long-term clarithromycin prophylaxis administered to 100 patients would be expected to prevent 27 cases of disseminated MAC over the median lifetime of the population at risk (36 expected disseminated MAC cases, minus 9 observed cases per 100 patients, assuming a median survival of 19 months). In a third, earlier macrolide prophylaxis trial, 693 patients with less than 100 CD4+ cells/μL were randomly assigned azithromycin (1200 mg once weekly), rifabutin (300 mg/day), or a combination of these drugs [24]. During the median follow-up time of 514 days, the incidence of disseminated MAC was significantly lower in the azithromycin group (13.9%) or the combination group (8.3%) when compared with that observed in subjects treated with rifabutin only (23.3%). Dose-limiting drug toxicity occurred in 13%, 23%, and 16% of the three stated patient groups, respectively [24]. Interestingly, the occurrence of macrolide-resistant MAC disease has been an infrequent event in the reported prophylaxis studies: only 2-3% of patients given clarithromycin and only 1% of patients given azithromycin suffered from an mycobacteremia with MAC isolates that became resistant to these drugs. In the year 2000, two randomized, controlled studies have compared azithromycin with placebo in patients with a CD4+ lymphocyte count increased to 100 cells/μL or more while on a potent cART treatment, and no prior history of disseminated MAC disease [3]. Specifically, in a study published by WM El-Sadr *et al.*, a total of 520 patients were enrolled with a median CD4+ count of 230 cells/μL at the time of entry. There were no cases of confirmed MAC in either the azithromycin arm or the placebo arm over a 12-month observation period [71]. In the other study conducted by JS Currier *et al.*, which enrolled 643 patients, only two episodes of MAC disease were observed among the 321 patients assigned to placebo, and no cases of MAC occurred among patients who remained on azithromycin, leading to an estimated incidence of 0.5 events per 100 person-years [72]. In both of these studies, the discontinuation of azithromycin prophylaxis was not found to increase the incidence of MAC disease significantly during a median of 12-16 months of follow-up, suggesting that it is safe to discontinue primary prophylaxis in those patients who achieved a significant CD4+ T-cell count recovery attributed to an effective cART regimen [72, 73]. With regard to *secondary prophylaxis* against MAC, in the earlist study evaluating the safety of discontinuing secondary prophylaxis for disseminated MAC, the investigators prospectively followed four patients with a known history of MAC disease. Antimycobacterial therapy was discontinued without evidence of recurrence after 8-13 months of follow-up [12]. Later, in a larger, prospective trial (JA Aberg, 2003), a total of 48 patients discontinued antimycobacterial therapy [13]. All patients had been on a macrolide-based regimen for at least 12 months, and on cART obtaining a CD4+ count of at least 100 cells/μL, sustained for at least 16 weeks. Of the 48 subjects, 47 remained free from MAC complications for a median of 77 weeks off therapy. One patient developed a localized MAC osteomyelitis 16 months after stopping secondary prophylaxis [13]. Concurrently, in a French retrospective study, three patients of 26 experienced a MAC relapse [14]: one of them was extremely immunocompromised (his CD4+ count was under 50 cells/μL at the time of relapse), and the other two individuals developed atypical bone infections, concurrently with a CD4+ lymphocyte count of 126 and 160 cells/μL, respectively [14]. In patients with increased CD4+ counts on cART, who develop atypical manifestations of MAC, it may be prudent to continue treatment for a prolonged period of 12-18 months, and then continue chronic suppressive therapy (secondary prophylaxis), for life. It is also critical to remember to re-start MAC prophylaxis if immunologic and/or virologic failure results in a decrease in the CD4 T-cell count. Presently, the absolute CD4 T-cell threshold indicating re-initiation is still debated, although the United States Public Health Service guidelines again recommend to consider a CD4+ lymphocyte count below 50 cells/μL, as a risk threshold to start antimicrobial prophylaxis. To conclude, in the cART era it appears sufficiently safe to discontinue antimycobacterial therapy in patients who have been successfully treated their underlying HIV infection, and achieved a sustained CD4+ T-lymphocyte count above 100 cells/μL for at least three months, and were previously treated with a macrolide-containing therapeutic regimen for at least 12 months.

Immune Reconstitution Inflammatory Sindrome (IRIS) and Atypical Mycobacteriosis

Presently, there is no unequivocal definition for the so-called "immune reconstitution inflammatory syndrome" (IRIS), and also the management strategies of this emerging condition are not uniformly agreed [74-77]. The IRIS syndrome tends to occur more frequently in individuals who are receiving cART for the first time (or after experiencing a prior therapeutic failure associated with a deep CD4+ lymphocyte depletion), and who experience a rapid decline in HIV viral load while on an effective cART [74, 77], associated with a concomitant, relevant gain in their CD4+ lymphocyte count. Although there have been some attempts to reach a better definition of IRIS based upon the entity of CD4+ cell increases and viral load reductions, the development or worsening of signs and symptoms soon after the initiation (or the re-start) of an effective HIV treatment (usually reported as early or paradoxical reactions), may also occur prior to the establishment of laboratory-based evidence of a quantitative "immune reconstitution", established on the ground of the absolute CD4+ cell count. Maybe, the most frequent and best described cases of IRIS have consisted of atypical manifestations just secondary to a latent-subclinical MAC disease in the setting of HIV infection treated successfully with cART [5]. This MAC-associated paradoxic clinical reaction produces an intense local inflammatory disorder against indolent MAC infections, in individuals given an effective cART, and experiencing an "explosive" and rapid increase of CD4+ lymphocyte count (and cell-mediated immunity as a whole). In the field of non-tuberculous mycobacteriosis, IRIS is manifested by painful suppurative lymphadenopathy, pulmonary infiltrates, and skin abscesses, usually associated with pleural and also abdominal effusion. A case report is briefly reported and depicted in Figure 1. As anticipated, IRIS has been reported more frequently among subjects who start or re-start a potent cART regimen in the setting of an acute or a latent opportunistic infection, occurring with an underlying, deep HIV-related cell-mediated immunodeficiency. From a management point of view, since IRIS usually results from actual growth of the opportunistic organism, a pathogen-specific therapy is always indicated. Antiinflammatory agents (usually non-steroideal antiinflammatory drugs, -NSAIDs-, buy also corticosteroids), may be of some benefit on individual basis, while it is still discussed whether a slightly delayed initiation of cART in patients which start a potent antimicrobial therapy for an AIDS-related opportunism may prevent or blunt the occurrence, the intensity, and the duration of IRIS signs and symptoms.

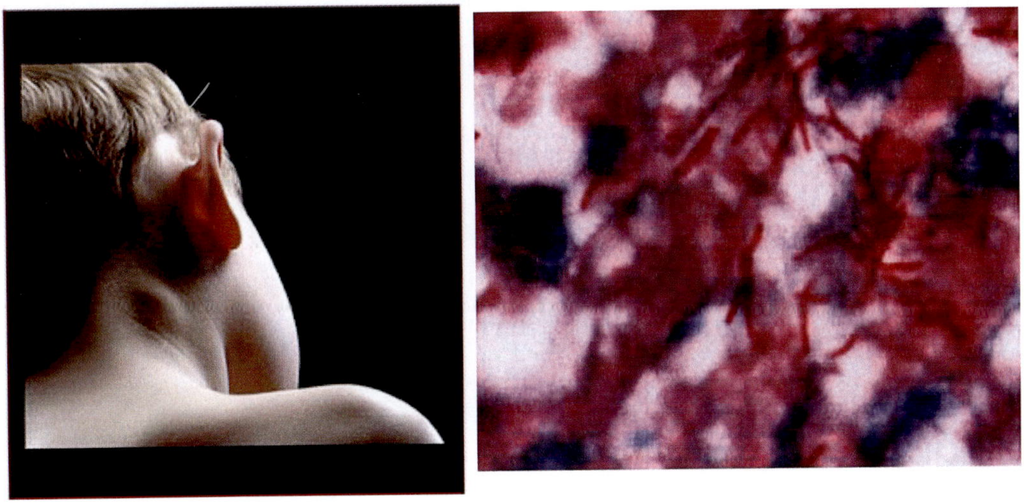

Figure 1. Immune reconstitution syndrome expressed by hyperpyrexia, fatigue, night sweats, bilateral pleural effusion, and multiple, enlarged lymph nodes, occurring in a HIV-infected patient who recovered over 200 CD4+ lymphocytes/μL after three weeks of a novel, effective cART regimen, started after failure and ascertained resistance to multiple, previous cART combinations. A lymph node biopsy disclosed a large amount of acid-fast bacilli, which were identified as *Mycobacterium avium* strains. Our patient already suffered from disseminated MAC disease, when 11 years before a diagnosis of full-blown AIDS was notified.

References

[1] Chaisson, RE; Moore, RD; Richman, DD; Keruly, J; Creagh, T. Incidence and natural history of Mycobacterium avium-complex infections in patients with advanced human immunodeficiency virus disease treated with zidovudine. The Zidovudine Epidemiology Study Group. *Am Rev Respir Dis.*,1992, 146, 285-9.

[2] Nightingale, SD; Byrd, LT; Southern, PM; Jockusch, JD; Cal, SX; Wynne, BA. Incidence of *Mycobacterium avium-intracellulare* complex bacteremia in human immunodeficiency virus-positive patients. *J Infect Dis.*, 1992, 165, 1082-5.

[3] Chin, DP; Hopewell, PC; Yajko, DM; et al. *Mycobacterium avium* complex in the respiratory or gastrointestinal tract and the risk of *M. avium* complex bacteremia in patients with human immunodeficiency virus infection. *J Infect Dis.*, 1994, 169, 289-95.

[4] Palella, FJ; Delaney, KM; Moorman, AC; et al. Declining morbidity and mortality among patients with advanced human immunodeficiency virus infection. HIV Outpatient Study Investigators. *N Engl J Med.*, 1998, 338, 853-60.

[6] Phillips, P; Kwiatkowski, MB; Copland, M; Craib, K; Montaner, J. Mycobacterial lymphadenitis associated with the initiation of combination antiretroviral therapy. *J Acquir Immune Defic Syndr Hum Retrovirol*, 1999, 20, 122-8.

[7] Sheppard, DC; Sullam, PM. Primary septic arthritis and osteomyelitis due to *Mycobacterium avium* complex in a patient with AIDS. *Clin Infect Dis.*, 1997, 25, 925-6.

[8] Miller, RS; Thomas, SJ; Hospenthal, DR; Oster, CN. Isolated *Mycobacterium avium* complex osteomyelitis in a patient with AIDS. In: Program and Abstracts of the 35th Annual Meeting of the Infectious Diseases Society of America; September, 13-16, 1997, San Francisco. Abstract, 574.

[9] Alisky, JM; Schlesinger, L. Isolated cavitary pulmonary *Mycobacterium avium* complex infection in a patient with AIDS. *Clin Infect Dis.*, 1998, 27, 1542-3.

[10] Hocqueloux, L; Lesprit, P; Herrmann, JL; et al.. Pulmonary *Mycobacterium avium* complex disease without dissemination in HIV-infected patients. Chest., 1998, 113, 542-

[11] Race, EM; Adelson-Mitty, J; Kriegel, GR; et al. Focal mycobacterial lymphadenitis following initiation of protease-inhibitor therapy in patients with advanced HIV-1 disease. *Lancet*, 1998, 351, 252-5.

[12] Shafran, SD; Singer, J; Zarowny, DP; et al. A comparison of two regimens for the treatment of *Mycobacterium avium* complex bacteremia in AIDS: rifabutin, ethambutol, and clarithromycin *versus* rifampin, ethambutol, clofazimine, and ciprofloxacin. *N Engl J Med.*, 1996, 335, 377-83.

[13] Aberg, JA; Yajko, DM; Jacobson, MA. Eradication of AIDS-related disseminated *Mycobacterium avium* complex infection after 12 months of antimycobacterial therapy combined with highly active antiretroviral therapy. *J Infect Dis.*, 1998, 178, 1446-9.

[14] Aberg, JA; Williams, PL; Liu, T; et al. A study of discontinuing maintenance therapy in human immunodeficiency virus-infected subjects with disseminated *Mycobacterium avium* complex. *J Infect Dis.*, 2003, 187, 1046-52.

[15] Zeller, V; Truffot, C; Agher, R; et al. Discontinuation of secondary prophylaxis against disseminated Mycobacterium avium complex infection and toxoplasmic encephalitis. *Clin Infect Dis.*, 2002, 34, 662-7.

[16] Chaisson, RE; Benson, CA; Dubé, MP; et al. Clarithromycin therapy for bacteremic *Mycobacterium avium* complex disease. A randomized, double-blind, dose-ranging study in patients with AIDS. AIDS. *Ann Intern Med.*, 1994, 121, 905-11.

[17] Koletar, SL; Berry, AJ; Cynamon, MH; et al. Azithromycin as treatment for disseminated *Mycobacterium avium* complex in AIDS patients. *Antimicrob Agents Chemother*, 1999, 43, 2869-72.

[18] Dunne, M; Fessel, J; Kumar, P; et al. A randomized, double-blind trial comparing azithromycin and clarithromycin in the treatment of disseminated *Mycobacterium avium* infection in patients with human immunodeficiency virus. *Clin Infect Dis.*, 2000, 31, 1245-52.

[19] Dubé, MP; Sattler, FR; Torriani, FJ; et al. A randomized evaluation of ethambutol for prevention of relapse and drug resistance during treatment of *Mycobacterium avium* complex bacteremia with clarithromycin-based combination therapy. California Collaborative Treatment Group. *J Infect Dis.*, 1997, 176, 1225-32.

[20] Sullam, PM; Gordin, FM; Wynne, BA. Efficacy of rifabutin in the treatment of disseminated infection due to *Mycobacterium avium* complex. The Rifabutin Treatment Group. *Clin Infect Dis.*, 1994, 19, 84-6.

[21] Benson, CA; Williams, PL; Currier, JS; et al. A prospective, randomized trial examining the efficacy and safety of clarithromycin in combination with ethambutol, rifabutin, or both for the treatment of disseminated *Mycobacterium avium* complex disease in persons with acquired immunodeficiency syndrome. *Clin Infect Dis.*, 2003, 37, 1234-43.

[22] Gordin, FM; Sullam, PM; Shafran, SD; et al. A randomized, placebo-controlled study of rifabutin added to a regimen of clarithromycin and ethambutol for treatment of disseminated infection with *Mycobacterium avium* complex. Clin Infect Dis., 1999, 28, 1080-5.

[23] Benson, CA; Williams, PL; Cohn, DL; et al. Clarithromycin or rifabutin alone or in combination for primary prophylaxis of *Mycobacterium avium* complex disease in patients with AIDS: A randomized, double-blind, placebo-controlled trial. *J Infect Dis.*, 2000, 181, 1289-97.

[24] Pierce, M; Crampton, S; Henry, D, et al. A randomized trial of clarithromycin as prophylaxis against disseminated Mycobacterium avium complex infection in patients with advanced acquired immunodeficiency syndrome. *N Engl J Med.*, 1996, 335, 384-91.

[25] Havlir, DV; Dube, MP; Sattler, FR; et al. Prophylaxis against disseminated *Mycobacterium avium* complex with weekly azithromycin, daily rifabutin, or both. *N Engl J Med.*,1996, 335, 392-8.

[26] Nightingale, SD; Cameron, DW; Gordin, FM; et al. Two controlled trials of rifabutin prophylaxis against *Mycobacterium avium* complex infection in AIDS. *N Engl J Med.*, 1993, 329, 828-33.

[27] Wolinsky, E. Mycobacterial diseases other than tuberculosis. *Clin Infect Dis.*, 1992, 15, 1-10.

[28] Kiehn, TE; Edwards, FF. Rapid identification using a specific DNA probe of *Mycobacterium avium* complex from patients with acquired immunodeficiency syndrome. *J Clin Microbiol*, 1987, 25, 1551-2.

[29] Yakrus, MA; Good, RC. Geographic distribution, frequency, and specimen source of *Mycobacterium avium* complex serotypes isolated from patients with acquired immunodeficiency syndrome. *J Clin Microbiol*, 1990, 28, 926-9.

[30] Tsang, AY; Denner, JC; Brennan, PJ; McClatchy, JK. Clinical and epidemiological importance of typing of Mycobacterium avium complex isolates. *J Clin Microbiol*, 1992, 30, 479-84.

[31] Crawford, JT; Bates, JH. Analysis of plasmids in *Mycobacterium avium-intracellulare* isolates from persons with acquired immunodeficiency syndrome. *Am Rev Respir Dis.*, 1986, 134, 659-61.

[32] Horsburgh, CR; Jr.; Cohn, DL; Roberts, RB; et al. *Mycobacterium avium-M. intracellulare* isolates from patients with or without acquired immunodeficiency syndrome. *Antimicrob Agents Chemother*, 1986, 30, 955-7.

[33] Hampson, SJ; Portaels, F; Thompson, J; et al. DNA probes demonstrate a single highly conserved strain of Mycobacterium avium infecting AIDS patients. *Lancet*, 1989, 1, 65-8.

[34] von Reyn, CF; Maslow, JN; Barber, TW; Falkinham, JO; Arbeit, RD. Persistent colonisation of potable water as a source of *Mycobacterium avium* infection in AIDS. *Lancet*, 1994, 343, 1137-41.

[35] Horsburgh, CR; Jr., Selik, RM. The epidemiology of disseminated nontuberculous mycobacterial infection in the acquired immunodeficiency syndrome (AIDS). *Am Rev Respir Dis.*, 1989, 139, 4-7.

[36] Winter, SM; Bernard, EM; Gold, JW; Armstrong, D. Humoral response to disseminated infection by *Mycobacterium avium-Mycobacterium intracellulare* in acquired immunodeficiency syndrome and hairy cell leukemia. *J Infect Dis.*, 1985, 151, 523-7.

[37] Wayne, LG; Young, LS; Bertram, M. Absence of mycobacterial antibody in patients with acquired immune deficiency syndrome. *Eur J Clin Microbiol*, 1986, 5, 363-5.

[38] Jacobson, MA; Hopewell, PC; Yajko, DM; et al. Natural history of disseminated *Mycobacterium avium* complex infection in AIDS. *J Infect Dis.*, 1991, 164, 994-8.

[39] von Reyn, CF; Barber, TW; Arbeit, RD; et al. Evidence of previous infection with *Mycobacterium avium-Mycobacterium intracellulare* complex among healthy subjects: an international study of dominant mycobacterial skin test reactions. *J Infect Dis.*, 1993, 168, 1553-8.

[40] Horsburgh, CR; Jr.; Mason, UG; 3rd, Farhi, DC; Iseman, MD. Disseminated infection with *Mycobacterium avium-intracellulare*. A report of 13 cases and a review of the literature. *Medicine (Baltimore)*, 1985, 64, 36-48.

[41] Wolinsky, E. Nontuberculous mycobacteria and associated diseases. *Am Rev Respir Dis.*, 1979, 119, 107-59.

[42] Iseman, MD; Buschman, DL; Ackerson, LM. Pectus excavatum and scoliosis. Thoracic anomalies associated with pulmonary disease caused by Mycobacterium avium complex. *Am Rev Respir Dis.*, 1991, 144, 914-6.

[43] Denis, M; Gregg, EO. Recombinant tumour necrosis factor-alpha decreases whereas recombinant interleukin-6 increases growth of a virulent strain of *Mycobacterium avium* in human macrophages. *Immunology*, 1990, 71, 139-41.

[44] Appelberg, R; Castro, AG; Pedrosa, J; Silva, RA; Orme, IM; Minoprio, P. Role of gamma interferon and tumor necrosis factor alpha during T-cell-independent and -dependent phases of *Mycobacterium avium* infection. *Infect Immun*, 1994, 62, 3962-71.

[45] Castro, AG; Silva, RA; Appelberg, R. Endogenously produced IL-12 is required for the induction of protective T cells during *Mycobacterium avium* infections in mice. *J Immunol*, 1995, 155, 2013-9.

[46] Newman, GW; Guarnaccia, JR; Vance, EA; Wu, JY; Remold, HG, Kazanjian, PH. Interleukin-12 enhances antigen-specific proliferation of peripheral blood mononuclear cells from HIV-positive and negative donors in response to *Mycobacterium avium*. *AIDS*, 1994, 8, 1413-9.

[47] Zakowski, P; Fligiel, S; Berlin, GW; Johnson, L; Jr. Disseminated *Mycobacterium avium-intracellulare* infection in homosexual men dying of acquired immunodeficiency. *JAMA*, 1982, 248, 2980-2.

[48] Wong, B; Edwards, FF; Kiehn, TE; et al. Continuous high-grade *Mycobacterium avium-intracellulare* bacteremia in patients with the acquired immune deficiency syndrome. *Am J Med.*, 1985, 78, 35-40.

[49] Nyberg, DA; Federle, MP; Jeffrey, RB; Bottles, K; Wofsy, CB. Abdominal CT findings of disseminated *Mycobacterium avium-intracellulare* in AIDS. *Am J Roentgenol*, 1985, 145, 297-9.

[50] Chin, DP; Hopewell, PC; Yajko, DM; et al. *Mycobacterium avium* complex in the respiratory or gastrointestinal tract and the risk of *M. avium* complex bacteremia in patients with human immunodeficiency virus infection. *J Infect Dis.*, 1994, 169, 289-95.

[51] Volpe, F; Schwimmer, A; Barr, C. Oral manifestation of disseminated *Mycobacterium avium intracellulare* in a patient with AIDS. *Oral Surg Oral Med Oral Pathol*, 1985, 60, 567-70.

[52] Blumenthal, DR; Zucker, JR; Hawkins, CC. *Mycobacterium avium* complex-induced septic arthritis and osteomyelitis in a patient with the acquired immunodeficiency syndrome. *Arthritis Rheum*, 1990, 33, 757-8.

[53] Cohen, JI; Saragas, SJ. Endophthalmitis due to *Mycobacterium avium* in a patient with AIDS. *Ann Ophthalmol*, 1990, 22, 47-51.

[54] Woods, GL; Goldsmith, JC. Fatal pericarditis due to *Mycobacterium avium-intracellulare* in acquired immunodeficiency syndrome. *Chest.*, 1989, 95, 1355-7.

[55] Cappell, MS; Gupta, A. Gastrointestinal hemorrhage due to gastrointestinal *Mycobacterium avium intracellulare* or esophageal candidiasis in patients with the acquired immunodeficiency syndrome. Am J Gastroenterol, 1992, 87, 224-9.

[56] Hawkins, CC; Gold, JW; Whimbey, E; et al. *Mycobacterium avium* complex infections in patients with the acquired immunodeficiency syndrome. *Ann Intern Med.*, 1986, 105, 184-8.

[57] Wallace, JM; Hannah, JB. *Mycobacterium avium* complex infection in patients with the acquired immunodeficiency syndrome. A clinicopathologic study. *Chest.*, 1988, 93, 926-32.

[58] Yagupsky, P; Menegus, MA. Cumulative positivity rates of multiple blood cultures for *Mycobacterium avium-intracellulare* and *Cryptococcus neoformans* in patients with the acquired immunodeficiency syndrome. *Arch Pathol Lab Med.*, 1990, 114, 923-5.

[59] Reves, R; Stone-Venohr, B; Hildred, G; et al. Utility of paired blood cultures in the diagnosis of disseminated Mycobacterium avium complex infection (abstract). In: Proceedings of the 8th International Conference on AIDS, Amsterdam, July 19-24, 1992. Amsterdam: Dutch Foundation, 1992, 127.

[60] Roberts, GD; Koneman, EW; Kin, YK. Mycobacterium. In: Balows A, Hausler WJ Jr, Herrmann KL, et al., eds. Manual of Clinical Microbiology. Washington, DC: American Society of Microbiology, 1991, 304-339.

[61] Shanson, DC; Dryden, MS. Comparison of methods for isolating *Mycobacterium avium-intracellulare* from blood of patients with AIDS. *J Clin Pathol*, 1988, 41, 687-90.

[62] Gazzola, L; Zanini, F; Zerbi, P; Franzetti, F; Gori, A. The usefulness of PCR assay in diagnosing disseminated mycobacterial infection in AIDS patients. *Eur J Clin Microbiol Infect Dis.*, 2008, 27, 163-6.

[63] Nichols, L; Florentine, B; Lewis, W; Sattler, F; Rarick, MU; Brynes, RK. Bone marrow examination for the diagnosis of mycobacterial and fungal infections in the acquired immunodeficiency syndrome. *Arch Pathol Lab Med.*, 1991, 115, 1125-32.

[64] Northfelt, DW; Mayer, A; Kaplan, LD; et al. The usefulness of diagnostic bone marrow examination in patients with human immunodeficiency virus (HIV) infection. *J Acquir Immune Defic Syndr*, 1991, 4, 659-66.

[65] Yajko, DM; Nassos, PS; Hadley, WK. Therapeutic implications of inhibition versus killing of Mycobacterium avium complex by antimicrobial agents. *Antimicrob Agents Chemother*, 1987, 31, 117-20.

[66] Yajko, DM; Kirihara, J; Sanders, C; Nassos, P; Hadley, WK. Antimicrobial synergism against *Mycobacterium avium* complex strains isolated from patients with acquired immune deficiency syndrome. *Antimicrob Agents Chemother*, 1988, 32, 1392-5.

[67] Fernandes, PB; Hardy, DJ; McDaniel, D; Hanson, CW; Swanson, RN. *In vitro* and *in vivo* activities of clarithromycin against *Mycobacterium avium. Antimicrob Agents Chemother*, 1989, 33, 1531-4.

[68] Inderlied, CB; Kolonoski, PT; Wu, M; Young, LS. Amikacin, ciprofloxacin, and imipenem treatment for disseminated *Mycobacterium avium* complex infection of beige mice. *Antimicrob Agents Chemother*, 1989, 33, 176-80.

[69] Cohn, DL; Fisher, EJ; Peng, GT; et al. A prospective randomized trial of four three-drug regimens in the treatment of disseminated *Mycobacterium avium* complex disease in AIDS patients: excess mortality associated with high-dose clarithromycin. *Clin Infect Dis.*, 1999, 29, 125-33.

[70] Kemper, CA; Havlir, D; Haghighat, D; et al. The individual microbiologic effect of three antimycobacterial agents, clofazimine, ethambutol, and rifampin, on *Mycobacterium avium* complex bacteremia in patients with AIDS. *J Infect Dis.*, 1994, 170, 157-64.

[71] Chaisson, RE; Keiser, P; Pierce, M; et al. Clarithromycin and ethambutol with or without clofazimine for the treatment of bacteremic *Mycobacterium avium* complex disease in patients with HIV infection. *AIDS*, 1997, 11, 311-7.

[72] Parenti, DM; Williams, PL; Hafner, R; et al. A phase II/III trial of antimicrobial therapy with or without amikacin in the treatment of disseminated *Mycobacterium avium* infection in HIV-infected individuals. *AIDS*, 1998, 12, 2439-46.

[73] El-Sadr, WM; Burman, WJ; Grant, LB; et al. Discontinuation of prophylaxis for *Mycobacterium avium* complex disease in HIV-infected patients who have a response to antiretroviral therapy. *N Engl J Med., 2000*, 342, 1085-92.

[74] Currier, JS; Williams, PL; Koletar, SL; et al. Discontinuation of *Mycobacterium avium* complex prophylaxis in patients with antiretroviral therapy-induced increases in CD4+ cell count. A randomized, double-blind, placebo-controlled trial. AIDS Clinical Trials Group 362 Study Team. *Ann Intern Med.*, 2000, 133, 493-503.

[75] Shelburne, SA; Visnegarwala, F; Darcourt, J; et al. Incidence and risk factors for immune reconstitution inflammatory syndrome during highly active antiretroviral therapy. *AIDS*, 2005, 19, 399-406.

[76] Lipman, M; Breen, R. Immune reconstitution inflammatory syndrome in HIV. *Curr Opin Infect Dis.*, 2006, 19, 20-5.

[77] Hirsch, HH; Kaufmann, G; Sendi, P; Battegay, M. Immune reconstitution in HIV-infected patients. *Clin Infect Dis.*, 2004, 38, 1159-66.

[78] Tuon, FF; Mulatti, GC; Pinto, WP; De Siqueira Franca FO; Grysheck RC. Immune reconstitution inflammatory syndrome associated with disseminated mycobacterial infection in patients with AIDS. *AIDS Patient Care STDs.*, 2007, 21, 527-32.

In: Cross Infections: Types, Causes and Prevention
Editors: Jin Dong and Xun Liang

ISBN: 978-1-60741-467-4
© 2009 Nova Science Publishers, Inc.

Commentary

Control of Emerging Infectious Agents Causing Nosocomial and Community-Acquired Cross Infections in Immunocompromised Hosts

Hossam M. Ashour
Department of Microbiology and Immunology
Faculty of Pharmacy, Cairo University, Egypt

Cross infection is the transmission of an infectious agent from one person to another because of a poor barrier protection as in patients and immunocompromised hosts. This can be a direct transmission or an indirect transmission through instruments, appliances, and surfaces. The most common are nosocomial cross infections, which are acquired at a hospital or other healthcare facilities such as outpatient clinics. Community-acquired cross infections have also been described.

Many of the microbes causing cross infections are resistant to antimicrobial agents and thus present a challenge in treatment and prevention. Examples include the traditional nosocomial cross-infection with methicillin-resistant Staphylococcus aureus (MRSA) and the recently characterized vancomycin- and linezolid- resistant Staphylococcus aureus isolated from hospitalized cancer patients [1]. The misuse of antibiotics might have contributed to the rapid evolution of vancomycin-resistant Staphylococcus aureus (VRSA) and linezolid-resistant Staphylococcus aureus strains in Egypt. This emphasizes the importance of sparing new effective antimicrobial agents and not using them routinely for the treatment of MRSA. An example of Community-acquired cross infections is MRSA isolated from inhalational and intravenous drug abusers, who could be a source or a reservoir of CA-MRSA infection in the non-addict population [2].

Cross Infection Control (CIC) is a term that encompasses all the measures taken to prevent the transfer of pathogenic microorganisms, which can potentially result in infection. Control of cross infections in a hospital, outpatient clinic, or a community setting is crucial, especially for immunocompromised patients, such as cancer patients and drug addicts [1, 2].

Unfortunately, the chain of cross infection control is easily broken when simple procedures are not observed. One important measure that is not adequately practiced by many healthcare workers is proper hand washing of healthcare workers, use of gloves, masks, and gowns, and compliance with strict hand hygiene guidelines and appropriate hand disinfection techniques [3]. It is noteworthy that the care of fingernails and the skin of hands are components of hand hygiene [4]. Healthcare practitioners who wear artificial nails are more likely to harbor pathogens on their fingertips than healthcare practitioners who have natural nails [5]. Wearing rings was also reported to increase the frequency of hand contamination with nosocomial pathogens [6].

Another CIC measure is to routinely examine the prevalence of MRSA and VRSA in different institutions and to strive to limit the introduction of antibiotic-resistant microorganisms into the health care institutions. This can be accomplished by efficient eradication of carriers and prompt physical isolation of patients who bear such organisms. A proper understanding of routes of cross infection is critical for CIC. A review of the literature revealed some modes of cross infection that are not necessarily obvious for some health care practitioners. Transmission of antibiotic-resistant microorganisms via the face is one route of cross-infection in hospitals [7] . Thus, hospital personnel must not touch their faces or elevate their hands above the shoulder in the ward, because many antibiotic-resistant bacteria can colonize the face. Pre-operative marking of immunocompromised patients with marker pens should also be very limited although disposable markers can be used, if necessary [8] . This is because marker pens can act as fomites for nosocomial infections. Beds, mattresses, curtains, and sphygmomanometers may be contaminated with micro-organisms. Surprisingly, the patient's own flora (carried intransally or elsewhere) can also result in nosocomial cross-infections of patients or non-patients with MRSA and other antibiotic-resistant pathogens [2].

All new staff members in a health care institution (a hospital or an outpatient facility) should be trained in accordance to the most up-to-date methods and procedures for infection control. The current staff should also be re-trained regularly. Auditing should be continuously carried to ensure the effectiveness of the procedure. The infection control protocols should be written and made available to the staff and the public.

A fundamental and motivating factor to CIC is self preservation, which is generated from the fear of becoming infected. Thus, raising the public awareness of the importance of the infection control measures will put an extra pressure on the health care staff members, which will make them more cognizant to the infection control measures. By practicing continuous efficient CIC measures, a health care institution will build up a reputation of safety and care for both patients and staff, which, over a period of time, can result in an increase in patients through recommendations. Time pressure due to a heavy workload might make some healthcare practitioners neglect some simple cross infection control measures. To avoid this, healthcare institutions should limit the number of patients that one healthcare practitioner could manage per day. Nonetheless, it will always be a personal responsibility for each member of the health care team to implement CIC consistently. Researchers should not only continue to characterize resistant microbes causing cross infections, but should also propose novel therapeutic and preventive approaches that could keep these infectious agents under control.

References

[1] Ashour, HM; A. el-Sharif, Microbial spectrum and antibiotic susceptibility profile of gram-positive aerobic bacteria isolated from cancer patients. *J Clin Oncol*, 2007, 25(36), p. 5763-9.

[2] El-Sharif, A; Ashour, HM. Community-acquired methicillin-resistant Staphylococcus aureus (CA-MRSA) colonization and infection in intravenous and inhalational opiate drug abusers. *Exp Biol Med* (*Maywood*), 2008, 233(7), p. 874-80.

[3] Tanner, J. Double gloving to reduce surgical cross-infection. *J Perioper Pract*, 2006. 16(12): p. 571.

[4] Boyce, JM; Pittet, D. Guideline for Hand Hygiene in Health-Care Settings. Recommendations of the Healthcare Infection Control Practices Advisory Committee and the HICPAC/SHEA/APIC/IDSA Hand Hygiene Task Force. Society for Healthcare Epidemiology of America/Association for Professionals in Infection Control/Infectious Diseases Society of America. *MMWR Recomm Rep*, 2002, 51(RR-16), p. 1-45, quiz CE1-4.

[5] McNeil, SA.. et al., Effect of hand cleansing with antimicrobial soap or alcohol-based gel on microbial colonization of artificial fingernails worn by health care workers. *Clin Infect Dis*, 2001, 32(3), p. 367-72.

[6] Trick, WE. et al., Impact of ring wearing on hand contamination and comparison of hand hygiene agents in a hospital. *Clin Infect Dis*, 2003, 36(11), p. 1383-90.

[7] Kuramoto-Chikamatsu, A., et al., Transmission via the face is one route of methicillin-resistant Staphylococcus aureus cross-infection within a hospital. *Am J Infect Control*, 2007, **35**(2), p. 126-30.

[8] Tadiparthi, S., et al., Using marker pens on patients: a potential source of cross infection with MRSA. *Ann R Coll Surg Engl*, 2007, 89(7), p. 661-4.

Index

A

B

C

D

E

F

G

J

K

L

Q

R

S